The Book of Heartfelt Moments
Book I

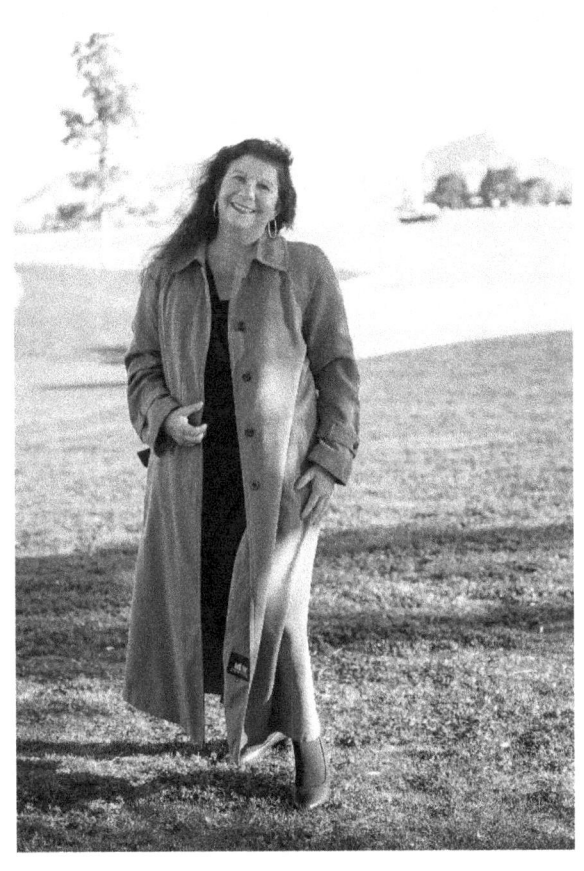

Susan Magestro

The Book of Heartfelt Moments Book I
Copyright 2024 © Magestro & Associates, LLC

All rights reserved. No parts of this publication may be reproduced, stored in a retrieval system, or transmitted in any form, or by means including electronic mechanical means. Photography and recording— without the prior written permission of the publisher is prohibited.

Table of Contents

Prologue 1

Part One: Inspirational People 4

Chapter 1: The Criminologist Comes Home 5

Chapter 2: Finding The People Who Look Like Me! 8

Chapter 3: The Silent Crusader 11

Chapter 4: She's Everyone's Daughter 13

Chapter 5: A Moment's Freedom 17

Chapter 6: A Victim No More 20

Chapter 7: Stability 23

Chapter 8: Better Off Together Than Apart 27

Chapter 9: Never Excuse Yourself 30

Chapter 10: Children Helping Children 33

Chapter 11: The 'Best-Est' Kindergarten Teacher 37

Chapter 12: Can One Point Change A Life? 41

Chapter 13: We Are Beta Sisters 44

Chapter 14: The Lost Thread 49

Part Two: Situational Inspirations 60

Chapter 15: Everyone Feels Like The Only One 61

Chapter 16: Truncated Grief 64

Chapter 17: Open Doors 67

Chapter 18: Circle Of Estrangement 69

Chapter 19: We Are Dedicated Professionals 73

Chapter 20: Who's Running Your House?" 76

Chapter 21: Averting The Shoot 80
Chapter 22: The Code Of Secrecy 84
Chapter 23: What Do Children With An Incarcerated Parents Look Like? 88
Chapter 24: Are You Afraid Of Your Child? 92
Chapter 25: Climbing Steep Mountains 95
Chapter 26: Waiting For The Normal 98
Epilogue 104

Prologue

Exactly three years ago, like everyone else, I felt the world had become a bad dystopian movie. I was ready for this movie to end. But it didn't. The world around me had changed. Suddenly, everything that I had previously experienced professionally, as a criminologist, was becoming part of our everyday lives. No longer was there a separation between what I experienced professionally and what I experienced personally. Every day behaviors were becoming paralleled to those behaviors I had witnessed in a prison. Suddenly, unacceptable, rude, and disrespectful behaviors were becoming commonplace. Anger, rage, and a lack of empathy were surrounding us. Violence had become a daily occurrence. I wanted so much to wake up from the nightmare that had become our lives. Quickly, I realized, this was more than a nightmare, it was becoming our new way of life.

The respect and character, so important to me to modulate my life as a criminologist had become 'watered down'. People all around me appeared complacent. Initially, many appeared non-plussed and oblivious to the new culture before us. Everywhere around me, I saw an increase in rudeness and an acceptance of just plain meanness. Bystanders appeared to be cheering it on; even applauding behaviors that became increasingly more insane. Previously, in my professional life, I had been able to walk away. I was able to keep grounded in my private life. Then suddenly, no matter where I went, the grocery story, the movies, driving down the street, Pandora's Box had opened. These new behaviors were becoming more outrageous and more people seemed to accept them, even found them funny and entertaining.

I felt compelled to change this, yet it was so much bigger than me. I came up with a plan that if I could find resilient people who have overcome adversity, just one at a time and celebrate them; I could fill myself up with positivity. Two years ago, I started writing about people I knew. They raised the bar so high. Their achievements moved me. Their resilience was so profound, all the while they maintained kindness and respect. I truly love and respect each of them.

Many of my friends loved hearing these stories as it filled them up as well. So, this is the story of twenty-five people and situations that moved me as the pandemic came to be the new normal.

I started printing these stories on Linked In. Through my analytics, I could see how many people were reading these essays and who they were by profession. Some called me, just to chat. Others would tell me, we follow your stories about life today and we'd like you to work with our professionals. Many said, "We can all identify with them." Others shared, "I thought I was the only one thinking about this". While some of these topics may be a bit bold, they are real. During this time of dystopian acceptance, I am moved to share these heartfelt stories that filled me up, at a time when our world needed a little kindness.

There are two parts to this book: Part One is written with a focus on people who overcame adversity to build resilience for themselves and those around them. Part Two focuses on situations to overcome these challenging times.

PART ONE
INSPIRATIONAL PEOPLE

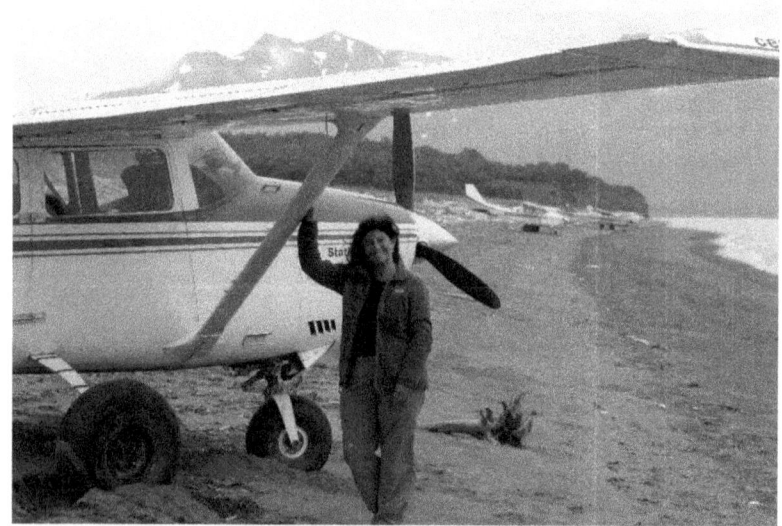

Nonna Off To Photograph Bears
We are never too old to follow our hearts.

Chapter 1
The Criminologist Comes Home

"A happy life consists not in the absence, but in the mastery of hardships." (Helen Keller)

I haven't been home in five years. I tried to come home many times over the last few years. I had the airplane tickets, packed my bags, but I couldn't make it to the airport let alone get on the plane. For decades, I have worked with horrific crimes involving children throughout the United States and internationally. I have been able to stay grounded and focused. But now, suddenly, life as I knew it was different. I now had PTSD. Why? A betrayal I had just experienced was so insurmountable, the violation of trust so unimaginable, I lost everything, except my life. I learned of a scheme perpetuated against an enormous number of women. It was horrific and unconscionable. I was faced with the gut-wrenching decision whether to disclose this unconceivable atrocity or focus on myself. You see, this time, I was NOT the criminologist working on a case, I was the casualty.

Five years ago, I was faced with a choice; leave my home and possibly survive, or stay home and be dead in months. It may seem like it was an easy choice, but it was by far the most agonizing journey of my life. Leaving and losing everything familiar went to a depth I did not realize would be as excruciating as it was. I thought I was tough enough to navigate it and walk towards the other side with honor, grace, and grit. That was not the case. Losing everything except my life brought me to my knees. I had to learn how to be grateful simply for my life, while also de-escalating the rage within myself. Most difficult, was trying to find forgiveness. Should appreciation for survival and some semblance of oneself be enough to forgive? I was forced to look introspectively whether the human spirit could survive losing everything except themselves and move forward? We see that every day now, don't we?

Upon being told I was going to die, due to taking a prescription, allegedly causing the deaths of hundreds of women, I knew all of my strength and healing had to come from deep within myself. I was encouraged to be the first woman to bring this egregious deceit to light. I searched for even a sliver of forgiveness at the start. I could not, even as a woman who has lived my life embracing forgiveness. I had to circumvent my thoughts that I would have gladly covered the cost of the pharmaceutical kickbacks this medical team allegedly received rather than be their guinea pig. Trying to block their scheme, they denied my referral to a leading research hospital as their actions could be revealed. I self-referred. For two years, I raged so deeply in my core, there were moments I wondered how I could ever feel peace again.

After finishing two years of treatment, I uncovered the "Dopesick" mentality of this scheme, unique mostly to rural states. I was threatened for this revelation. Initially, I acquiesced to stay quiet. I healed, grew stronger, and continued my work as a criminologist, but I was never the same. My spirit felt almost dead. I was sure it was.

Today, with the embrace of my dear friend of forty years, I got on that plane, then drove five -hours home finding the peace I never thought I would find again. Early on, I told myself I was tough, my journey was another bump in the road, and I would persevere. Intrinsically, there were many moments I questioned this. I had lost my familiar, my home, my family and friends, incurred astronomical debt, and fought for my life in a way I had never fought for anything; mentally, physically, or spiritually.

Today, five years later, never really certain the day would come, I came home. I took the boards off my home and dream of a trauma retreat for first responders and front liners. It had taken me twelve years and every spare hour and dollar to build this dream. The majestic snow- capped mountains and glistening blue waters of the inlet were so powerful that I wept away the rage I had built up for five years. Now, I feel at peace, a goal of overcoming PTSD. Now, I embrace my dreams for my future; one I never thought I would have. Little did I know that taking the boards off this beautiful trauma retreat, meant for my colleagues in breathtaking Homer, Alaska, would be just what I needed to help overcome my own trauma.

I took a warrior pose on the deck overlooking the blue waters and snow-capped mountains. I could breathe for the first time in five years. Can you come home again? I think you can. I fought like hell to get here.

Chapter 2
Finding the People Who Look Like Me!

"Faith is taking the first step even when you don't see the whole staircase." (Martin Luther King)

The text came to me late on a Monday night. "I'm not sure if you can help me with this or if you are still investigating but, I need to find someone." She signed her name. Remembering her well, I reflected to the time when she was 13 years old; strong, determined, and very angry. She was a foster child placed in the system when she was 6 years old by a mother who later reclaimed her other siblings, but not MW. She never understood why she was forced to remain in foster care when her siblings were not. The number of her foster home placements was unimaginable with the conditions equally so. MW looked at other kids and was repeatedly saddened that other children had a family to celebrate milestones and special moments, but she did not. It pulled at my heart as she told me this story decades later, much as it did before.

MW turned the unbearable and relentless rage she felt within, into becoming an amazing athlete who stood out in her community. People came out just to watch her, even if they weren't affiliated with her school. MW became a local celebrity adored in the news. She was unstoppable, winning a college scholarship on the other side of the country. After graduation, she went into a career that promises to protect and serve. She also became a foster parent herself.

Now in the fourth decade of her life, she still had no idea of who her biological father is but knew this was the time to find him. MW had received results from popular genetic testing sites that she had just participated in. She was overwhelmed with the content which seemed like a foreign language along with disjointed connections, few of whom she knew. Unclear where to begin or how to navigate all this, she reached out to me. I told her I would walk along side of her, not as investigator but as a friend, explaining how to gather and analyze the information she found. The plan was for her to reach out to 5-10 contacts a day, put the information on a sticky note on the wall, then we would analyze all the information she gathered. We made plans to connect in a week and strategize the next move.

Three days later, MW called me with such joy and elation in her voice, "I found them in just three days! I am part of a family!" she exclaimed. "I found my family!"

We went over every detail. In just three short days, she emailed many people on her "genetic list". She decided to look into the background of one in particular that indicated they were half siblings. She found her sister on social media. Immediately, MW called the school where her sister was a teacher. Even though it was during the school day, the secretary unknowing the reason for the call, patched it through to a landline in the classroom that her sister was covering, for a short while. MW heard her sister's voice for the first time and it sounded familiar. With great trepidation, she shared, "Uh, I am your half -sister. I just found you." Her sister dropped the phone and screamed. All the students in the room asked what was going on and in the next few moments they all shared in the re-connection of these lost siblings.

It has now been eight days since MW reached out to me. Not only has she connected with sisters, brothers, aunts, and uncles, she has a plane ticket to meet with them just twelve days after her phone call to me. Bittersweet, she learned that her father passed away a year ago and he never knew about her. One of her aunts sent MW a picture of her father. "I look like him. This is my family." Her late father's ex-wife called her to welcome and embrace her into the family. What grace MW felt from this unexpected call. The upcoming reunions planned with her new- found family are sure to be what movies are made of.

"I found where I belong," she cried in joy and I cried with her, feeling so blessed that this girl reached out to me. I am grateful I was able to be a small sliver in her journey. MW really gave me a gift, filling me up through her pure and raw joy. This heartfelt moment will resonate with me for the rest of my days. I will end this story with the way we ended every phone call, "Cool beans!"

Chapter 3
The Silent Crusader

"Yes," she thought laying down her brush in extreme fatigue. I have had my vision." (Virginia Woolf)

BB could be the person next to you at the store, the person you see walking down the street or standing next to you at Starbucks. Today is her 80th Birthday. BB is one of the finest women I have ever known. She has been one of my strongest role models. The smile in her voice has always made me feel so welcome and grounded. Her strength resonates to all who have had the good fortune to know her, even when they are low. You'd never know her age. She is beautiful, strong, resilient, and has a 'bee-bop' to her step that few can keep up with. BB has had such a tremendous impact on tens of thousands of young people and their families.

She has this type of magnetism; I could listen to her speak for hours and never feel like I have heard enough of her stories. She is humble and wise, a combination rare these days. To the tens of thousands of young people, she has impacted, to the professionals who were fortunate to learn from her, the happiest of birthdays to a woman who knew a secret many will never know; meet people where they are, not where you are.

She reached out to the most high- risk of our young people and created programs that they had to strive to get into, stay in, and achieve. Almost all, rose to that expectation never wanting to disappoint her. Because of BB, these once high risk youth could grab a future they could be proud of and attain their personal dreams. BB believed in them, truly moving mountains to create realistic ways that THEY could attain their potential, even with the challenging realities that were their lives. Those fortunate to have come into her world, happily traveled hours each day to make sure they showed up to complete the programs she personally created, so each of them could achieve their potential greatness. They never wanted to not let her down. And in the end, they became our airline pilots, international renown chefs, translators, mechanics, and more. They learned to be accountable; at first to her, and then to themselves, what a rich life lesson.

She is a woman who created rainbows for countless young people. Because of her, we see them all around us thriving today! Happy Birthday BB-what a legacy you have created. I am one of the lucky ones because you are in my life.

Chapter 4
She's Everyone's Daughter

"Hello darkness my old friend, I've come to talk with you again," (Simon and Garfunkel)

I remember with great clarity, the moment I learned my friend's daughter, Jordyn, and my former student, had been killed by a drunk driver. She was walking to the store with a friend, to shop for school supplies; anticipating the start of school, the next day. They were on the sidewalk. I knew I must have misread this article; distracted by a medical emergency within my family. Sadly….I did not misread this article.

I remember absolutely every detail of the last time I saw Jordyn. I didn't just see her, I felt her. We were exploring future careers that might be of interest in her future. She looked at me with her sweet blue eyes and beautiful, shoulder length copper hair. "What type of career gives you a little spark?" I leaned down to ask her privately, smiling at one of my kindest students.

She looked back up at me with her saucer shaped eyes and softly said, "I can't say, I really don't know," with such sweetness. That was Jordyn. She just didn't know or did she? I made a mental note to come back around and revisit that with her again. We never did.

The driver was coming from a social event which included an afternoon of drinking. He failed to navigate the curve or modulate his speed. Life changed in a split second; just one moment in time. That day, Dayna, her family and our community, lost the life of one of our sweetest innocents. Many of my friends who are first responders were called to the scene that day. It was one of the most difficult 'call outs' many of them had ever experienced and they worked hard to cope. It felt like Jordyn was everyone's child and the grief was palpable. That feeling never left as we all tried to put one foot in front of the other to walk alongside this mother, this father, our friends, our neighbor.

The pain for this precious family seemed unimaginable, unfathomable, and so very unfair. Somehow, they had to dig deep, to the center of their cores, for strength as they had two other children. My friend, Dayna, explained that her pain felt like a deep burning, like a fire that just would not stop. There was nothing, there was no one who could put out this fire. While this immense pain has never left Dayna, she recognized her heart was divided; one third of her heart was in a state of unrelenting torture, believing the only way she could move forward was to go be with her daughter. Two-thirds of her heart had to hold strong and maintain for her children who were still alive and struggling as well.

We all stood with Jordyn's family; feeling like she was your daughter, my daughter, our daughter. Immediately, she became everyone's daughter. While we all remember the details of that awful day, we have chosen to replace those by embracing all that was so beautiful about Jordyn, believing she lives on within us forever.

Jordyn's amazing mother, Dayna endured an agonizing horror we privately pray will never visit again. Yet, in her unimaginable grief, my friend, Dayna held up, not just for her daughter, her boys, her husband, and her family; she stayed strong for everyone else's child, not once but twice!

A few weeks before Jordyn was killed, her mother had just been promoted from teacher to a new assistant principal of a school that specialized in students who needed 'just a little extra'. In her enormous grief, Dayna returned to work after two weeks, to make sure everyone else's child was able to navigate their first weeks of school. She knew those early weeks set their foundation and ability to acclimate for the remainder of their entire school year. Intrinsically, this gave Dayna the purpose to keep moving.

At the sentencing hearing for this drunk driver, Jordyn's parents presented a series of pictures for the judge's consideration so he could know their daughter. The pictures were challenged and the agony of now prolonged hearings and trials continued. All thought this would be the finality, but it was not.

There was yet more for this family to endure. During those days, Dayna suspected the unrelenting headaches, fatigue, and blurry vision she was experiencing was as a result of the massive stress and heartache. She never had a moment's relief.

There was more to come. Further testing, evaluations, and diagnosis revealed there were still more mountains for this family to climb. Dayna was diagnosed with a brain tumor. During the agonizing diagnostic procedures, Dayna heard Jordyn close by telling her sweetly, "You will be ok, mom. God and I am here with you." Dayna could feel her.

It has been ten years since Jordyn was killed and eight years since Dayna's successful surgery. During every one of those years, Dayna has continued to support your child, my child, everyone's child; so, they can walk on the sidewalk with the 'gitty anticipation' of buying their school supplies for the start of the new school year. Dayna is not done giving back. While not a club she would have chosen membership, Dayna wants to continue to stand by parents who have lost a child, so they know they are not alone in their grief. Until the day when she is once again with her sweet Jordyn, Dayna makes herself available so other grief stricken parents can see their will be light one day.

My friend Dayna…. it is my privilege and a humbling honor to call her friend. She is one of the people in my life who gives me pause, always mindful of the importance of a moment. Days after Jordyn's death, she was sitting in her room crying. Her precious eleven -year old son told her, "I'll be strong for you mom." Today, he is now an adult and living a life of service to make a difference in the lives of others.

My life is richer today because of Dayna, her family, and the foundation they have created for families facing a similar tragedy. She continues to remind me that showing one's feelings is a sign of strength and humility, not a sign of weakness.

Chapter 5
A Moment's Freedom

"If wrinkles must be written upon our brows, let them not be written upon the heart. The spirit should never grow old." (James A. Garfield)

Nadine is a woman I consider memorable and striking. Once you see her, you never forget her. She is statuesque, a lifetime runner. She has a kind face and warm eyes. "Talk to me," is written on her forehead and everyone does! Her smile is wide from ear to ear; giving you the security that everything at this moment feels like it will be okay. She just turned sixty but you would swear she could not be a day over thirty-five.

At a quick glance, or for those who do not know her well, her life seems like a light, smooth breeze. Some have even said she is someone to be envied. In some ways that is true. Nadine has touched the lives of more children than anyone can possibly count, always encouraging them to stay away from drugs, live a healthy lifestyle, and be all you can be. She is spiritually grounded which she shares openly. Her artwork, as well as her style of speaking, is always with such purpose. I take a deep breath after listening to her and savor her tone and words within. I believe her enormous identity comes from her deeply connected Native roots. These are just a few things that move me deeply about her.

Unless one knows Nadine well, they would never imagine how tethered she has been for decades; sometimes by choice and sometimes by no choice of her own. Nadine has raised three grandchildren and has been her son's third party custodian for numerous criminality charges. Sometimes, he had to be within her sight and sound for up to a year at a time. This meant she could never leave the house without him or travel more than a ten -mile radius from the house he was calibrated to remain in. Working remotely, and shifting to running on a treadmill inside, instead of the outdoors she loved, permitted her to carry out the commitment she took on. She loves her son unconditionally. No outdoor running, no impulsive trips to the store, no doctor's appointment, no meeting with friends, no going out for a drive, or going out of town overnight. She carried out the oath she took to the court, no exception ever!

Nadine started raising her oldest granddaughter at the time of her birth since her son and daughter-in-law's incarceration. This was followed by revolving doors filled with parole violations. That has been about twenty years now. Nadine raised her granddaughter to be a truly lovely young woman. Grandma was acutely aware of the challenges this child would face if grandma didn't stand by her side. Then, over the course of years, there were more grandchildren born to her son, with different mothers. She loved each of them, raising each to be fine and upstanding little people.

How does a sixty -year -old woman commit her life to raising three grandchildren, within a fifteen year span, giving up the dreams and visions she had for herself as she entered the later season of her life? Her friends are traveling, planning for retirement, and living the dreams they set out for themselves. Nadine is attending kindergarten conferences, packing school lunches, and helping with homework. She remains unflinchingly positive. Her strategies are brilliant because they are tangible and available.

To Nadine, her faith gave her the center to always believe everything would eventually be alright, even as it was falling apart around her. She explained that it was her running; the physical exercise that allowed her to stabilize and re-center her mind. She has made it a point to surround herself with only positive people who have supported her and the children, without judgement. She's had her small core of friends and a loving family who understood her choices; it's about the children.

She wasn't going to walk away from those children for someone else, perhaps a stranger to raise. She wasn't going to let these children enter a foster system that could haunt them for the rest of their lives.

She's sees the positive moments and milestones in each of their lives; celebrating each of their accomplishments as they are climbing their mountain. And when she needs a little getaway, she stands in the sunshine and sees positivity in all they do and who they are becoming.

This wasn't her plan for this time in her life, but it's how it turned out. She is surrounded by children who love her and know of the love she has for them. At the end of the day, she is clear and stands strong …..she can't imagine her life any other way. And when she dies, she knows, she will have lived the richest of lives, surrounded by all the little hands, now all grown up.

Chapter 6
A Victim No More

"The weak can never forgive. Forgiveness is the attribute of the strong." (Mahatma Gandhi)

She knew her grandfathers would dance with her at her wedding. Unfortunately, that was not to be, as they had both died before she married her wonderful man. She took pictures of her grandfathers and put them in a locket she wore as a bracelet. That way they were close by her as she walked down the aisle. Her new husband's uncle, who he was very close with, was not to be at the wedding either, as he had passed away as well. Lory took the picture of this wonderful uncle and put his picture into her groom's cufflinks. His uncle was going to be very close to him on this special day.

It was a spectacular day! To bear witness to a young woman I have come to love for thirteen years now. There are moments I feel like she is a daughter. She knows, unequivocally, the meaning of grit. So many times, when she did not see, I was moved to tears celebrating the profound woman she has evolved into. Anyone else would have been filled with hate, but Lory chose life; to live life and to love life. We all have a lesson to learn from her.

I saw Lory before I met her. She walked on the stage, her voice quivering, "My name is Lory," she began. The room was quiet even with over five hundred people in attendance. I decided to listen to her before I approached her not wanting to scare her off. The anxiety she must have been feeling to tell her story for the first time was palpable to all.

Thirteen years ago, just before this young woman celebrated her first adult birthday, she endured an unfathomable horror. She was stabbed more than seventy-six times throughout her body outside her school during the lunch break. A passerby saw the crime happening. He called 911 then intervened. He too was met with the knife. Helicopters circling, Lori relied on all her inner strength not to pass out. She willed herself to stay present, to stay alive. She endured surgeries, and painful healing beyond our imagination. Lory's scars from this egregious attack were apparent on the outside but I knew the depth of those types of scars on the inside.

Just one month later, she walked right back into that school where she had been attacked, greeted her friends and teachers, like it was just another day. I often ponder, who did she do that for, herself or for those traumatized around her?. I know the heart of this woman and I believe it was for both.

Given the option to finish her senior year at home, she boldly refused, walking for graduation with her life -long friends. She never let those around her know of the unrelenting pain she was in from the healing of more than seventy–six stabbings. While she fought hard and persevered, most who cared for Lory at this time would not have guaranteed she would have survived. She did more than survive, she thrived. She didn't live life as a victim, she lived a life she'd always wanted, that of a strong woman.

The details of this dark and grisly crime have become a little more buried, a little less important as time has gone on. It is the woman who refused to become a victim who will always be celebrated in my heart. The details of her crime should not be what is mesmerizing or fascinating. The celebration is to honor the strength and grit it took for Lori to evolve into a loving young woman and wife she has become.

After the ceremony, her handsome groom surprised her with a helicopter ride, uniting them as one. They flew off to a mountain pass, just the two of them. The mountains, like Lory, have weathered the most challenging of storms. They reawaken glorious and powerful, as they continue to grow.

The bride and groom had their private moment to celebrate her survival, their love, and their future. Then they climbed back into the helicopter, returning to their guests to celebrate the rest of their lives.

Chapter 7
Stability

"I raise up my voice-not so that I can shout, but so that those without a voice can be heard."
(Malala Yousafzai)

How does a mother continue to provide stability for her child after her husband is gunned down in front of them? Sadly, I have two women in my life who have had to address this gut-wrenching question. Both women were able to raise fine, fine sons; giving them insurmountable and unwavering stability even in the depths of their own fragility.

One of these mothers held her husband in her arms moments after he was shot by a stranger on a shooting spree right in front of her at the entrance of a restaurant? What horror she must have felt when the shooter then walked down the street headed in the direction of her only child? I cannot imagine what those moments must have been like for my friend. She and her child survived. How did she maintain sanity and stability to be able to raise her child even in the throes of such unfathomable tragedy?

One of my long time, special friends…her husband was gunned down in front of their home as he was opening the garage door. Their two sons were waiting and watching from inside the car. My friend dedicated her life to raising two fine sons. She also went on to make a difference in the lives of absolutely every child living in her country. She is lovely, graceful and strong. One would never know of her tests or the fortitude it took to be so very magnificent. She continues to be one of my most special friends.

Both women were tenacious, holding on to stability in the face of trauma. Both offered their children (as well as themselves) the ability to not only survive, but eventually thrive. I have thought about this a lot in the last few weeks as I am getting to know my new friend and missing my old friend. Respect. That is what I feel for both of these mothers.

Stability during trauma takes more than enormous strength, it takes grit. What crossroads my friends faced. Both mothers and their children were dealing with grief, trauma, and the justice system, all while trying desperately to maintain stability. Stability because life went on.

We know stability is one of the most important components of raising a child. When a child is raised with consistency and strong parenting they are better able to absorb the challenges they will face in their lives and climb the mountains they will find in front of them. In time, prioritizing stability in the throes of trauma will allow a child to continue to live a life safe to explore curiosity, safe to retain what they are taught, and safe to develop the confidence to explore their own lives, their own truth, and their own future. Stability in the face of trauma will allow these children to modulate their emotions and attitudes which in turn affects not just those around them; it affects all of us. They have a better chance to develop to their full potential rather than crumble into a pool of mud; which they may never get out of.

Maintaining stability for our young people is on shaky ground, more now than ever before. Meeting our children's basic physical and emotional needs must constantly be recalibrated as it is forever changing; never allowing for a parent to be complacent. Trauma is around most of us right now, often hitting a little too close to home. As parents and professionals, we must be cognizant that anything less than providing stability and consistency right now invites challenges further down the road.

We hear about crime, but seldom about how a family fights hard to survive and rise up when they are faced with unfathomable tragedy. And rise up they did! My friends grieved, stayed focused, and were committed. Are they still grieving? They tell me that perhaps a piece of them always will.

Stability has provided the grounding to allow them to heal one day at a time. A deep faith in God and a sense of honor to help others has continued to allow them to move forward with hope and forgiveness. For one, it is seventeen years and for another, it is over twenty years. Their smiles light up the room. Their voices have such strength and conviction. The joy in their hearts is shared with those around them. The sadness that comes in waves, they have learned to modulate within. Every day that I have contact with my two friends, be it in person or online, is a good day. Both have lived their lives with inspiration and passion, always reminding others of what is important during these challenging times. They took it one day at a time focusing on the stability that was needed to allow their surviving families to thrive.

Today, both of these mothers and all of their children make a positive impact on so many in their communities and their countries. The strength exhibited by both of these women, have made a lasting place in my heart-always.

Chapter 8
Better Off Together Than Apart

"Saying farewell is also a bold and powerful beginning." (Aron Ralston)

It was October of 1989 and I was enjoying a singles group, in San Diego. I didn't really talk to IG much, but a friend of mine had asked me what I thought of him. I said well, he seems a little too skinny for me and that was the end of our conversation. Two months later, I moved into my condo. I was in the middle of unpacking when that same friend called. She invited me to go to a party. I really didn't want to go, I wanted to finish unpacking. She begged me, "I don't want to go by myself". I agreed to go for a little while and threw on some leggings and an oversize sweater, definitely not dressed up.

I met IG again and we spoke for hours. He told me about another event the following weekend. I was non-committal. Smiling, he told me if I didn't agree to attend, he was going to come and pick me up. Of course, I went! The following weekend, we went on our official first date for his favorite, pizza. We saw each other pretty much every night from that point on.

Five weeks later, he got down on one knee and asked me to marry him. I said yes and nine months later we were married. That was one year to the day after my San Diego trip, when my friend asked me about the man I thought was too skinny. Fourteen months later, we welcomed our first daughter into the world and went on to have three kids in four years. Our family was complete.

Daddy time began each afternoon when he came home. He would sit in the middle of the living room and the kids would run around him in circles as he'd reach out and grab them to give them each a big hug and kiss. This game became known as "run around daddy". Lucky for us, he also knew his way around a kitchen. On Sunday mornings, he would put on a chef's hat and transform into "chef dah-da". The more he embellished his own unique chef accent, the more the kids giggled and laughed.

We truly enjoyed our children and although funds were tight, they recently told us they never felt deprived or that they were missing out. IG had a great imagination and there were plenty of things that could be done on a budget and be quite enjoyable.

While our children were our priority, we always made sure to make time for us. This included date nights.

We had a very strong foundation. Although we had our moments where we were at odds with each other, we always knew we were better off together than apart and always worked out whatever differences we were having. We complemented each other in some areas, while our values aligned perfectly in others. We had the same goals and planned for an amazing future together.

Unfortunately, sometimes, life has a way of altering those plans. IG passed away after a courageous battle with cancer. We are grateful for the years we did had together. We were blessed to have the foundation that makes a relationship last; a deep respect and friendship that lasted throughout our lives together.

Chapter 9
Never Excuse Yourself

"Never underestimate the power of dreams and the influence of the human spirit. We are all the same in this notion: the potential for greatness lives within each of us" (Wilma Rudolph)

"Work harder than anyone ever expects of you and never excuse yourself."

"Teens, if you can't get yourself out of bed and you don't put effort into anything, that is who you are going to be for all your life."

"Basketball is your vehicle,' her mantra to her players.

"Practice now for the adult you want to be!"

These are the words spoken by a magnificent woman who has been my friend for almost forty years. What an inspiration and role model for young women. I first met DB when I was facing a hard decision whether to make a career change that was in the best interest of my family, but meant trading one passion for another, along with an enormous pay cut.

When I met her, I was instantly greeted by a woman who exuberated honor and integrity. I came to call her style "athletic panache". Where did she buy such cool suits? Her world was made up of All Americans, ESPN, and USA Basketball. To this day, she says what she means and means every word she says. There's no BS, she just 'keeps it real'. She's efficient and her hands reach wide.

Frequently featured nationally as high school coach of the year, she is the epitome of holding the bar high for youth, as well as adults around her. People work hard to rise up, so as not to disappoint her, remaining there until it becomes intrinsic within themselves. Even as they have grown into adulthood, those whose lives she has touched, stay in touch with the woman they know 'sincerely gave a damn about them'.

"I like to think I help people see the possibilities in themselves, in a multitude of ways," she says. DB has carried her philosophy deeper by helping others who didn't have another way to see things for themselves, to believe in themselves and their future. Here we are now, forty years later as grown women of yet another season.

We have navigated the waves of major illness, job changes, births and deaths of family and friends, retirement and un-retirement, still returning to what we love several times now; making a difference in the lives of those around us. Now, late in our lives, she has taught me how to perfect the art of keeping desert dust off furniture and floors.

More importantly, DB has taught me that even as we age, there is always another peak waiting, even if it appears different than we would have imagined. Because of DB, I still continue to look at possibilities in a different way. She is one of my biggest supporters and I am hers. She has taken what I thought was our 'efficiency' to yet another level. As I make another important decision in my life, she has walked along side of me.

In my decades of working in a field that is both curious and torturous to many, there is not a moment I have lacked purpose. My friend has helped me to realize that my purpose, while still strong, may take root in another way. Stepping back from front line investigations, I embrace the opportunity to teach and pass on the techniques and strategies I have developed to professionals today. Like DB and I, these professionals work every day to bring clarity, balance, hope, and safety to our young people and their families.

We raise the bar high, show them how to get there, and remind them to never forget being accountable. I am so fortunate to have the kind of friend I can laugh with, cry with, fall down and get back up with. Without saying a word, she has lead by example. In celebration of the upcoming Thanksgiving Holiday, I want to say I am so thankful for DB and for the countless professionals who give of themselves, selflessly to make a difference in people's lives every day.

Chapter 10
Children Helping Children

"There is no real ending. It's just the place where you stop the story." (Frank Herbert)

The mudslides were enormously devastating, leaving many young children orphans. The year was 1998, the location was the Costa Rican/ Nicaraguan border.

Two things happened the following year. An ex-pat from South Dakota, Irv Whilheit, offered the families who lived on his land and worked for him in Costa Rica, a rewarded opportunity to adopt some of these young children thus making them part of their families. Many did, dozens of children were adopted. Irv and the community embraced these new arrivals.

The young children made quite a trek to school each day, crossing the Inter-Americana Highway. One morning, several of the adopted children, all in 'grade kin-der' were hit by cars and killed.

During that same time, a woman who goes by Su, traveled to Costa Rica as many as six times a year from Alaska. She saw friends and worked cases that were not often talked about.

That same year, when Su returned to Alaska, she found herself in an atypical situation. Su had to really think outside the box in order to connect with students who had become hardened to the struggles in life. She was standing in front of this group and remembered the children in Costa Rica trying to readjust to their new lives and losses. She told her Alaska students about them. That seemed to move them in a way she had not predicted or seen before. Without giving this idea a lot of deep thought or planning, she blurted out, "Let's build a school for these children."

The next day, the students entered their classroom and told Su they couldn't stop thinking about this story. They had told their parents, their families, friends and within one day, they devised a plan. They would tell the story of the orphan children throughout the USA and run a penny drive. This actually turned into a lot more than pennies!

Instantly, they became academically motivated in all their classes, to meet Su's requirements of C's or higher in all classes to participate. She had not planned all this out ahead of time, it seemed to have a life of its own! Many of the students went to second hand clothing stores to buy new clothes since they were now on television. Their project became news worthy.

The idea became a reality in full swing and lasted for about six weeks. Senators from Washington DC, grandmothers from Texas donated. Traffic was back up for miles every morning as lines of cars waited to drop their accumulation of coins to the students and teachers waiting out front with oversized watercooler jugs. The students, along with teachers, took shifts each morning. Over $75,000 was raised during those weeks. Local news channels caught wind of this story, reporting the progress regularly. It became a popular story.

Each student in the class had a task and they had to figure out how to work together. They became friends; their idea and dream became a savored reality. After the funds were raised, Su traveled down to see Irv again. He donated the land for the small school and Su's students raised the money. Together Irv and Su oversaw the construction of this building. They were in absolute awe; children helping children across the Americas. Both sides benefited from this project and for many, it changed the trajectory of their lives.

This merger went together much more smoothly than one might expect. The school was created with retractable walls between the classes looping the grades, 1 /2, 3/ 4, and 5/ 6. And of course there was a class for 'kinder'. This way the building doubled as a community center in the evenings and weekends.

Before the digging began, the people in the town greeted Su, who was joined by her own young son. They were met with a celebration of fried fish, other delicacies and a bottle of Coca Cola. After a wonderful meal, all joined hands, forming a big circle around the area that was to be the new school; photos were taken. Irv had remembered a prior conversation Su had shared with him hoping to one day find a conch shell from the beach. Still in a circle, several of the children came to present her with a conch shell they had found at a nearby beach as a thank you gift.

Today, almost twenty-five years later, the Alaska students, now all grown up, tell Su about their own dream; to one day take their own sons and daughters to see the school they had a part in building.

Irv has recently passed away in Costa Rica at the age of 99 years old. His community near Playa del Sol lives on. And today, as 2024 comes to an end, Su has celebrated this incredible memory. She has passed the conch shell on to her youngest grandson, the son of the son who was with her that day. It fills her with joy to think one day, her grandson will one day visit the school, and pass down the meaningful story behind the conch shell as well.

Chapter 11
The 'Best-est' Kindergarten Teacher

"Under pressure, the most important thing I have to remember is to breathe." (Curtis Strange)

There is no pain greater than watching your child struggle through the impossible. As a parent, you bargain, you make promises if only you can absorb their pain; just let their pain go away. Anything for the pain to be yours instead of theirs.

For Monica that was not to be. When her daughter was ten months old, this single mom and college student had her strength put to the test. Her baby was flown out of state, half a continent away for open heart surgery. What seemed to be the fix turned out to be temporary. Later, her young daughter was diagnosed with trachea-esophageal fistula, terminal for most babies as they drown in their own saliva. How did her young daughter survive this? No one could answer that nor did any of the medical professionals understand how the baby learned to cough in order to clear her throat, usually an impossibility for other children diagnosed with this.

This was not the end of their story. As she grew into childhood, her daughter was frequently hospitalized in ICU for weeks at a time. Every time this small young family thought they had turned the corner or reached the end of 'this road', they had not.

Monica finished college and went on to become my 'absolutely favorite kindergarten teacher'. I have met wonderful kindergarten teachers in my decades training educators, but Monica was always different to me. At the beginning, I did not know about her daughter.

Everyone loved her, whether they were her students or not. Parents loved her. Her staff loved her. Me, I loved her for a totally different reason. It is often said that a kindergarten teacher knows. They can predict and identify a student's future lifelong struggles at the young age of five or six. Monica was an absolute master at this. She not only identified these kiddos, she did everything within her power to turn behaviors, to compensate and teach children (and their parents) another way. She was gifted; making each of the children feel like they were special. They felt her unconditional love and worked hard to please her.

I spoke with Monica often during her tenure. She identified, observed, and lovingly chartered what was needed to turn those students in her charge. Because of Monica, the trajectory of many lives has taken a promising path, for her students as well as their families. She made these changes not only for her students, but for other children, other families, and others in the communities. For some, not as fortunate to walk with such a magnificent kindergarten teacher, their lifetime struggles continued. Her strategies, always offered with consistency, love and firmness, were embraced, acknowledged and appreciated. It wasn't just the message, but the approach as well as the delivery.

I met Monica when her daughter was entering middle school. From the moment I first met her, I thought she was beautiful. Her presence made you smile. Her cheerful eyes lit up her face always saying 'I'm so happy to see you". She brought such peace to others. Little did many know of her own private struggles with her own child; a little girl who was her heart.

Towards the end of high school, her daughter started having unexplained abdominal pain. It seemed to come on randomly after an eight -year hiatus. Monica thought they were finally seeing the light at the end of the tunnel. Once again, her daughter started to go downhill and change. Pain will do that to a person. Her daughters' physical pain and mental anguish was insurmountable for the young mother to watch.

Nonetheless, Monica continued to negotiate for her daughter's wellness, which was not to be. Again, and again, in and out of ICU. In order to work and survive, Monica had to compartmentalize the agony she was experiencing with her own child and step into the lives of little people. For many, she was the best part of their day. No one knew of the brevity she was struggling to contain, except those closest to her.

It was around this time that Monica's daughter realized she was different than the other kids and might always be. The young family still did not have a definitive diagnosis. Friends dwindled as the young girl couldn't commit to plans. Monica started to intrinsically worry, "What will happen to my daughter when I die?" She couldn't go to college, it was a struggle to finish high school being in so much pain. She couldn't hold a job. Just so many couldn't-s.

Monica knew she had to do something. This was the turning point. She took her daughter to PALOM for one month. It is a center where they explore dual diagnosis. Medications are synchronized and clients learn coping skills to live with their chronic pain.

Fast forward to today. Monica's daughter has her own apartment, close to her mom. Her daughter navigates each day with a positive attitude, thankful she can now do the little things for herself. Monica is now married to a supportive partner, enjoying her life in ways she didn't have space for before. But now both she and her daughter have found a new normal that works for them. Her daughter feels empowered by the little things she can now do for herself.

Monica, my very favorite kindergarten teacher has touched the lives of hundreds of young children, and because of that, there are thousands more she will never know. She has provided foundation for them to soar, much like the foundation she provided for her own daughter. She loved them all and kept them close in heart. Now she is retired, still young, still beautiful and inspirational. She still has the sparkle in her eye and that dimple when she smiles. She has a lift in her step. Monica, the 'bestest' kindergarten teacher, now has time for something she has never had time for…..her beautiful self!

Chapter 12
Can One Point Change A Life?

"Always remember: silence and a smile are two very powerful tools." (Paul Coelho)

Can one point negatively change the trajectory of a person's life? We all know it can. The real end to the story is not about the missed point, or the immense loss, but about how a person moves forward, circumventing malice and cruelty to achieve their best life regardless.

One of the professions I always hold in highest regard are educators; teachers, principals, counselors, school secretaries, and janitors. I am in awe of their hearts, their drive, and determination to make a difference in the lives of their students. Their profession is a life choice; often following their passion or calling. The challenges they continue to face are enough to cause most people to run. They stand rooted; role models of strength and possibilities.

Most educators struggle to motivate students they believe have potential but are under-achievers. Their professional reach to help 'mold and create the future' is powerful and lifelong. Today, I met a rare find; one who appears to have a track record to try to destroy those most aspiring. I am disappointed to bear witness to one who tried to destroy a high achieving, hard-working graduating senior two weeks before graduation.

This student had achieved excellent grades; attended a year and a half of college while a junior and senior of high school, along with becoming a "second in state athlete" in her sport, all the while working two jobs to make ends meet. Her family was strong in spirit, not affluence, and thus this student walked a path she set out early in life, cognizant of the realities of achieving her life dream to be a nurse anesthetist.

Two weeks prior to graduation, a teacher informed this student she may not be graduating because she may not be passing a class she had previously achieved a collegiate grade of B for, when she completed this in a prior college class. All were aghast as this young lady has always been a focused student with strong grades, all work turned in, no unexcused absences, never a behavior issue, respectful, etc.

Two days prior to graduation she was given a thumb's up, 'she could walk during graduation', however, now that the teacher had caught up with her "grading", the student's end grade was a 69%. The student offered to submit extra credit and was denied. Those close to the student met with the teacher, counselor, and administrator, raising concerns why this wasn't caught sooner, why suddenly extra credit was not available, especially when this student was one of the school's website posting achievers, for both academics and athleticism. The teacher, counselor, and principal were informed this one point would cost this student the academic scholarship she had worked so hard to achieve at a university she always dreamed of going to. They would not relent. A background check into this teacher revealed she has consistent history of selecting a few students from each of her classes, usually those most quiet, and ridiculing them in front of the class, telling them to go sit down and figure out how to work the calculus formulas from You Tube. Her ratings published online are very low by many who have taken her classes for these reasons.

This young student lost her academic scholarship due to this one point. She will still persevere. She will still attend the combination bachelor/master's program she has strove to be accepted to. How will she pay for it? She will continue working two jobs, take out loans, and she will have 'her best life' in time. This young lady has incredible depth and strength. She also has a heart of forgiveness. I am happy to report this student is soon to graduate with her degree in nursing and has already been accepted to move forward with the graduate portion of her program.

I am sure if the teacher and student's path's cross again one day, 'this now nurse,' will provide her patient nothing short of excellent care; because one point may change the path, but it will not alter the dream.

Chapter 13
We Are Beta Sisters

"Today is the oldest you've ever been and the youngest you will ever be." (Eleanor Roosevelt)

How do six women from different parts of the country; from the east coast, all the way to Alaska come together! In spite of their vastly different backgrounds, these women have come together to become friends collectively? I have had the gift to know each of them well at different times in my life. Now they have grown into a group of friends that has made their collectiveness all the richer.

They met for the first time just a little over a year ago. Who are they?

I will start with SG, I have known her all my life. She is one of the most beautiful women I have ever seen; with dimples, the kindest of eyes and a smile that radiates to all around her. My memories of her are vivid and rich, her voice has such lift and joy. There have been times I have called her with nothing much to say. I just love hearing her voice. I call her our Princess Bride. Yet, it is her spice and unsuspecting adolescent rebellion that continues to keep us giggling. We have shared many challenging and important moments from the time we were children to today. SG lives in CT. She is a brilliant interior designer with a flair for color and patterns. She can turn a love seat ever so slightly to capture a whole new ambiance in a room. She has dedicated her spare time to working with pet rescues and adoptions. Watching classic movies is her passion. I am the lucky one to be able to call her cousin.

SP was one of my best childhood friends, meeting when we were just five years old, living just a few houses apart. She lives in PA, is a counselor and mindfulness specialist. Reconnecting as adults, we did not miss a beat, laughing about our off-key rendition of Blowing in the Wind during a middle school talent show. She patiently practiced cartwheels and jerkies with me for cheerleading tryouts. She made Captain and I was picked last on a squad of twelve. Her encouragement allowed me to achieve that childhood dream. I cherish the moment we shared making second cuts for the boy's baseball team at a time when girls were limited in their choice of sports. The strongest vision I hold of my best childhood friend, SP, is when we were fourteen. I looked outside the back of our station wagon as our family drove away from the childhood home I adored to gallivant around the United States. We drove for three months until my family found the right place to settle. Every one of those days I thought about waving goodbye to my best friend. But that was not to be the end of our friendship as we picked up where we left off. She is wise, thoughtful, strong, and independent. She looks exactly the same; beautiful. Memories of our childhood friendship still warm my heart.

MA has been my dear friend for over ten years. She lives in MN, is a master social worker and now principal working every day with issues that tug at our heart. Consistently, respectfully, and without judgement my friend shows never ending grace and strength. She finds joy in the moments that 'exceed expectations'. For many, she is the best part of their day. Her smile is contagious and her eyes enormously genuine. She has worked and studied along -side me in many states; flying five hours to celebrate the one hundredth, final conference I would ever put on again. Even with hundreds of people in an audience, MA stands out. She has so much depth which has enabled her to provide a calm grounding for others to lean on. I am thankful every day that she and I have each other to lean on. We are so deeply interwoven, we can finish each other's thoughts. MA and I are so rooted and grounded in our connection that we reach out to each other because we can 'just feel it' when the other is having a challenging moment. What a gift MA is in my life. I can only hope everyone has a friend like her!

DE is a one of my most special heroes. She has enormous inner strength and resilience; overcoming what a bestselling novel is made of. Escaping into the dark and recreating a new life for herself and her children was just the beginning. Then she dedicated her professional life to helping children, so marginalized, few want to take on the task. She has created such a peaceful surrounding, I love to go and just be in the space she has created. While we are sometimes over 10,000 miles apart, we have learned to replace dinners at our favorite restaurant with planned wine nights and phone chats that last for hours. Most importantly, it is DE who showed me how to create gardens special to each of my grandchildren, filling us with a lifetime of laughter and fun. We met at a door more than twenty-five years ago. She was walking in and I was walking out. For all this time, that door never closed again.

KW is a friend that shows more and more of her inner grit every time we come together. We met sampling Argentinian Appetizers and knew we'd be friends. The friendship was solidified the day I realized I forgot to pack my black pants on the night I was to present at a special celebration. I forgot my backup black dress as well. Both uncharacteristic, but understandable, I was chasing major deadlines, planning a huge event and navigating a family emergency; all of which left me totally depleted. Giving myself one last look in the mirror with a sigh, I left the bathroom running toward the stage, feeling frazzled and less presentable than I ever felt before. As I left the bathroom, KW grabbed me, adjusted a little here and there. Then she said, "You look great, now go up there!" She instinctively became the strength and stability I needed at this most exhausting moment. My new friend KW. As we have peeled back the layers of our lives, I am in awe. Her rebound and long recovery from an unexpected and frightening health emergency is one you'd never suspect as she moves with flair and style. Imagine my delight as I had the pleasure to watch her 'bust out on the dance floor' at a recent event. Deep inside that did not surprise me at all! Another evening, we beamed when we saw each other. I had just recently cut a lifetime of waist length, long, thick black hair to a shoulder length. She knew what no one else did, it was about so much more than simply cutting the hair. It was about the liberation and all we do to get there. My friend KW, we walk that path arm in arm.

These are the women who have come together with me as our Beta Reading Team. They have read all of these Heartfelt Moments, as well as the endless re-writes of my two new books. Every other Monday night, we have met virtually for an hour or two. Exhausted from a long day and the promise of a busy week, we still made time for each other. We have been doing this now for almost two years. And when we finish Beta Reviews, we visit and talk about the impact of life today; adding our collective wisdom. This group of accomplished women became friends, not just with me, but each other. They became friends virtually for years, until they met, just fifteen months ago.

It was an enormously moving experience for me to watch as they hugged and visited and laughed like old friends. It was as if they had known each other for a lifetime; yet they had just met. What a thrill to be able to watch them.

Until we all come together next time, I want them to know that individually and collectively, I not only adore them, but I respect and cherish them in my life. My life is deeper and richer because of the sisterhood in my life. Thank you, Beta Sisters!

Chapter 14
The Lost Thread

"Always be the best you can be, for yourself, not for others. Don't dress to please others. Don't act to please others. Live authentically, Shoo. Live you and love you." Elgee Bove

In one split second, you can open a box and it changes your life. It did mine.

"Did you know about your uncle?" wrote a distant relative whom I had recently connected with?

Of course! I knew the man I still called Uncle Honey, even when I was twenty-five years old. I knew he was engaged to Ginger from Gilligan's Island. I knew my uncle was a famous dress designer.

Yet in reality, I discovered I didn't know all there was to know about Elgee Bove. As I learned more, I realized I could move forward in two ways; I can be sad about how ostracized he was despite his remarkable accomplishments, or I can celebrate a remarkable life that never got his familial due. I chose the latter.

In these last two years, I have been blessed to learn who my uncle really was. He was discovered by Judy Garland when he was in the twelfth grade. She was so taken with his gifted fashion designs that she hired him immediately. Ms. Garland discovered he was a child prodigy, who never had a fashion design class, and attended a high school in a neighborhood where most students didn't graduate. He designed her own personal wardrobe as well as the remake of costumes for her Broadway show. Before the age of eighteen, she brought him into the circles of MGM.

Opening this door further, I learned he earned over a million dollars a year, starting at nineteen years old and his hands were insured with Lloyds of London for over $100,000 in the 1950's and 60's. He was voted the youngest and most successful American Theatrical Designer in the United States, not only winning national awards, but honored by President Eisenhower for outstanding business success, an inspiration to the youth of the United States.

Soon thereafter, he started his own line of clothes designing for Marilyn Monroe, Evita Peron, Jayne Mansfield, Ava Gardner, the Gabor Sisters, and so many others. When MGM was trying to change the image of Jayne Mansfield to be more scantily clothed, he spoke up on her behalf.

He designed clothing for women with the motto that clothes do not make the woman, the woman makes the clothes. He believed that while clothes can make a woman feel beautiful, it is most important for her to feel beautiful within herself. He did not believe women should dress just to please a man. His ground-breaking campaigns for Revlon with Dorian Leigh, and later with Jessica Biel, were wildly popular back then as well as today. He was ahead of his time campaigning for women, even before the 1960's.

Bove's creations are everywhere, bolero jackets, boas, strapless dresses. His original clothing line, Salbert and Elfreda is now known as Elfreda. His fashions and designs can be seen on the internet and he is written about on numerous sites.

I grew up being told he was a 'loser'. That breaks my heart and the shortsightedness of these comments are clear presentations of dramatic familial lore.

Even with all the accolades from others and enormous wealth early in life, Elgee Bove died alone, and without the respect of his family. Very few family members who judged him met him maybe once or twice in their lives. Instead inaccurate stories were passed down by the generations. He was incredibly worldly and savvy. Some in the family considered him odd.

I have great memories of him setting up a miniature easel, just for me, right next to his. This went on until I was about six years old. He frequently re-stocked my own personal supply drawer. I remember I brought a smile to his face as he looked over at each of my creations. I constantly reminded him I was creating a fantastic replica of his mastery. He would fill me with kisses, hugs, and we would make funny faces at each other. I saw him throughout my childhood, until we moved away. I was fourteen years old. Then suddenly, I did not see him again until I was twenty-five.

Now, I can't help but be a little heavy hearted. My Uncle Honey, I didn't know he was such a gifted 'child prodigy' revered by the public. These incredible accomplishments were never shared by his family. I learned of this well after his death. Would it have mattered? Absolutely! How can a compassionate, sensitive, and accomplished man be so ostracized by those closest to him. I knew his primary focus was to bring out the inner beauty in others? I would have adored standing by his side through the ups and downs had I known.

I still remember well, a night when I wore the simple off the shoulder black dress he designed. "I want a woman to feel beautiful wearing my dresses." I did feel beautiful standing in his creation. I thought of him often at the Gala in the Captain Cook Ballroom. He was so intrinsically kind and so multi-talented. Many of his qualities have been passed down to my children and grandchildren.

Discovering this has been surreal. Why would so many of the accomplishments of such an amazing man of such inspiration to others, be kept a secret? Was it an eccentric flamboyance that put off some closest to him. Regardless, it is unconscionable to me that a parent did not celebrate this child. My uncle was cast out by those who should have loved him the most. I am still perplexed by this today.

To commemorate his authenticity, and achieving so much greatness, we enthusiastically planned a celebration of life for El Gee Bove the same year I opened the box and found his creations. This extraordinary celebration was filled with music, photos, a show of his replicated designs, lots of food, family, and friends. I hope my Uncle Honey looked down at us that evening; smiling as he will now live on, for generations to come.

Little did I know, we had so much more to come. The mysteries and realities of the life of this famous dress designer, have now been investigated and uncovered. Few knew who he really was. Internationally, he was declared missing during the mid- 1960's. But to me, his Shoo, he was never missing. I saw him often during this time of our lives. How perplexing that was to me initially, missing yet he was with me.

I have learned the famous dress designer was the front for who and how he actually lived his life. There is so much more to his life and loves. Who better to uncover the mysterious life of this fashion icon than his niece the criminologist. His ultimate sacrifice and love was for our country, which will be shared in a novel to be released in 2025. I do have a publisher.

All the times we sat across from each other…the world believing he was dead or missing. Our lives paralleled so very, very much. Yet, we did not speak of investigations, we did not speak about crime. Instead, we spoke about the way to approach people, the way to carry ourselves in various situations, the way to smile with your eyes and your heart and still steer the conversation in the direction you need to, sometimes difficult but always authentic.

I would have loved to have the opportunities to have long conversations with him about our "other" work. So today, who better to uncover the real life mysteries of Elgee Bove than his niece, the criminologist.

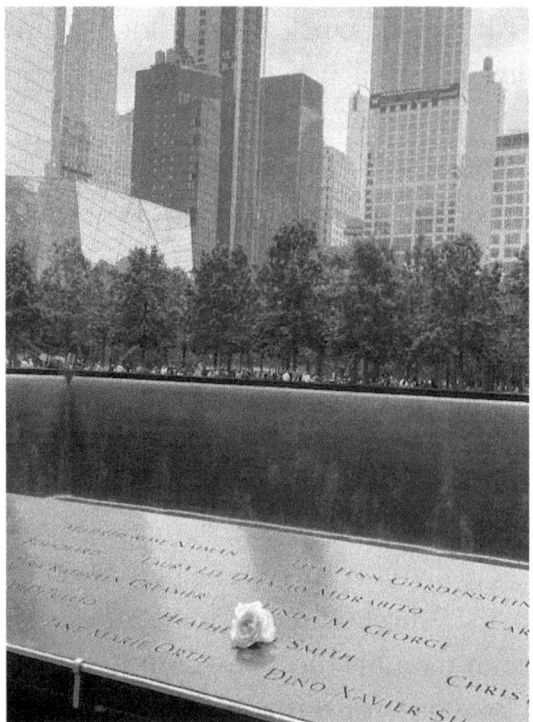

911 Exhibit. Never forget.

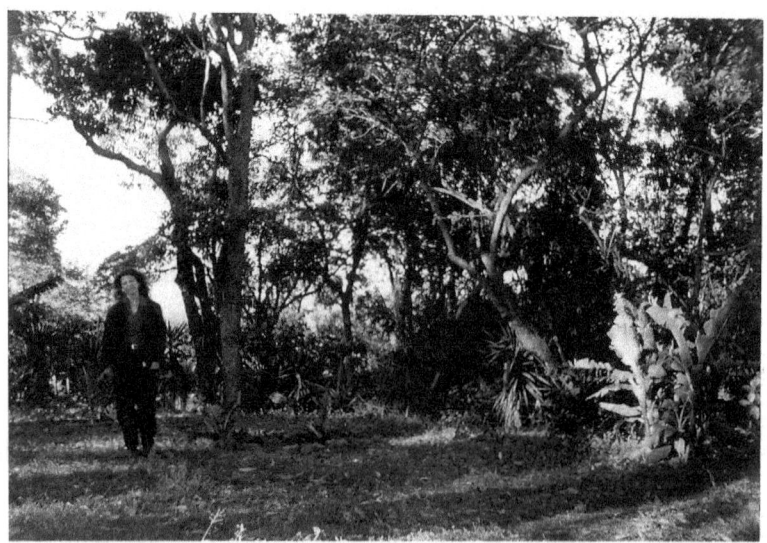

Rebirth. Each of us have our special moments of rebirth
Hold those images close at heart.

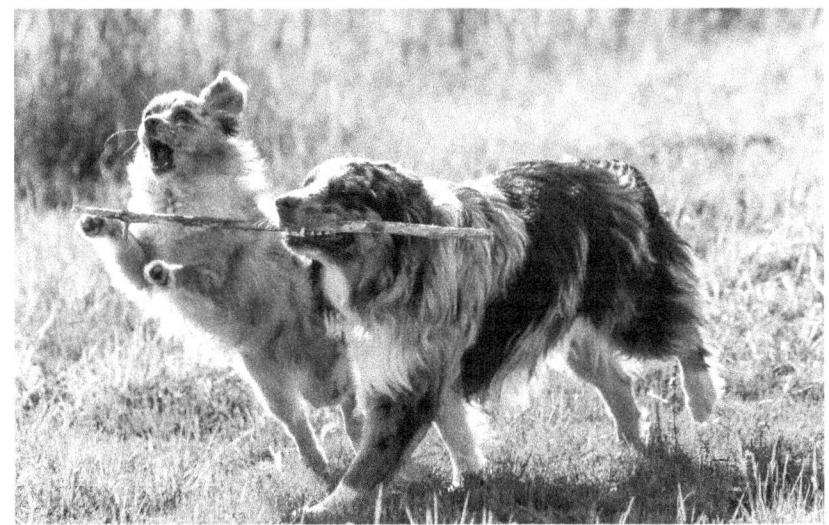

Keeping Up: Our dogs are a huge piece of my life. We were a family of Labs and Shebas. We are now totally enamoured with all our Mini-Aussies!

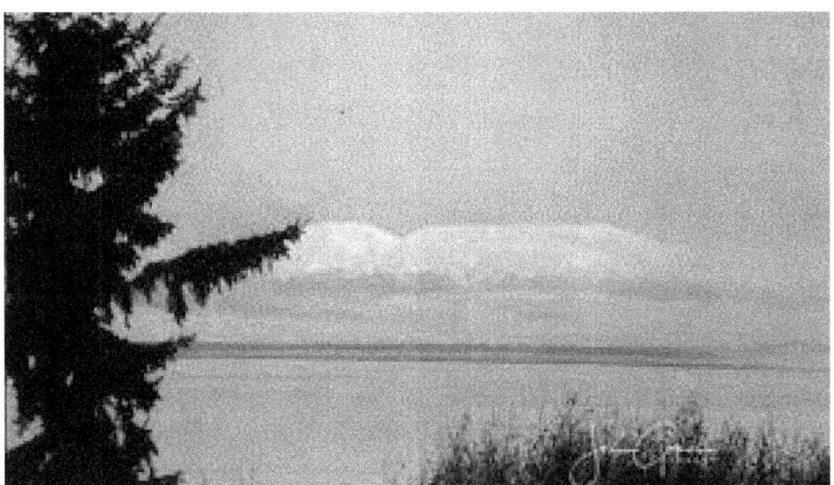

Sleeping Lady. When life is overwhelming, I speak to the Sleeping Lady.

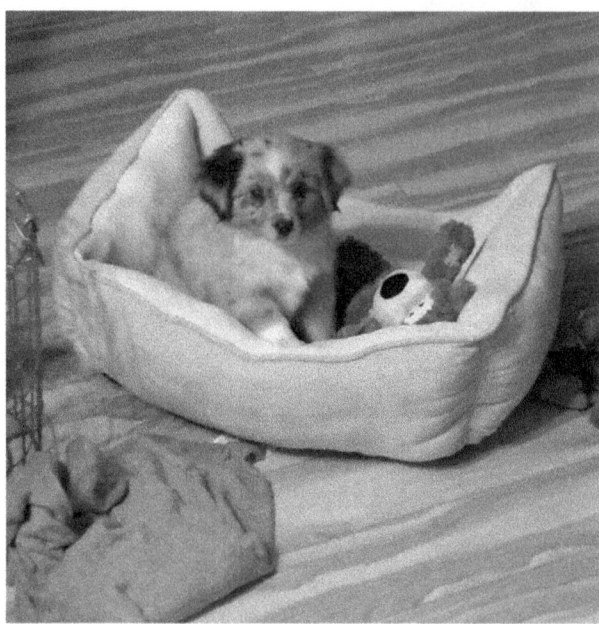

I Love Lucy. Lucy, my trauma, crisis dog. The plan was for her to work with me on my cases. Instead, she became my trauma dog; when the criminologist turned into the casualty.

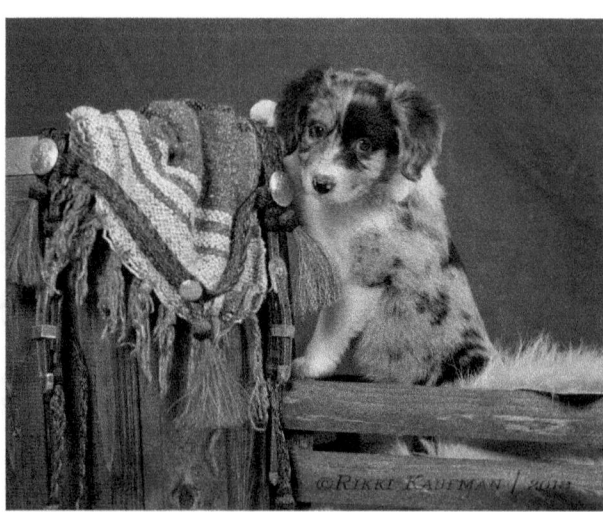

My Leap of Faith. Sometimes, timing may not be the best. Sometimes, others do not understand your decisions. The girl we call 'Kindness', my 'leap of faith', taught me to always remember, it will be okay.

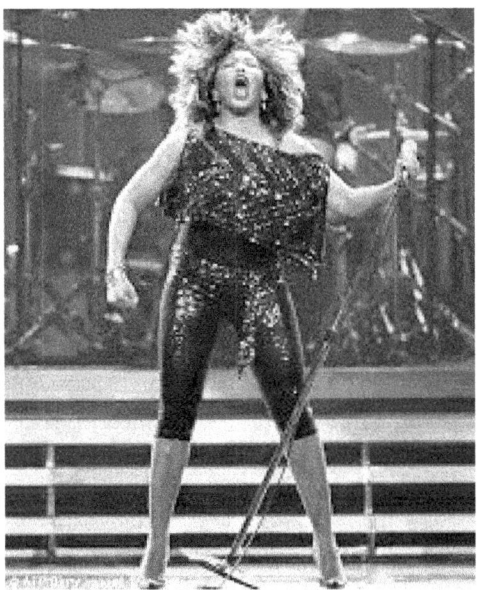

My Hera. It was my Hera, Tina Turner, who led me through the two most excruciating days of my life.

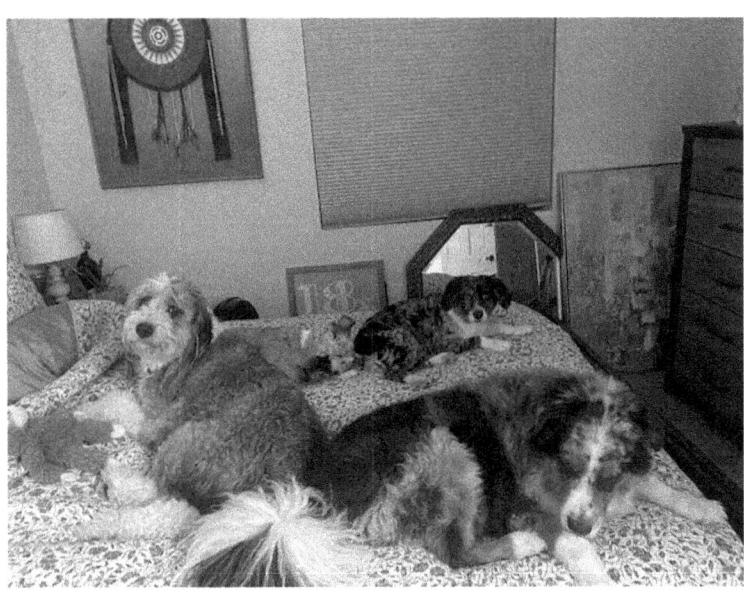

Aussie Sleep Over. Just to fill up with pure joy. Is there room in the bed?

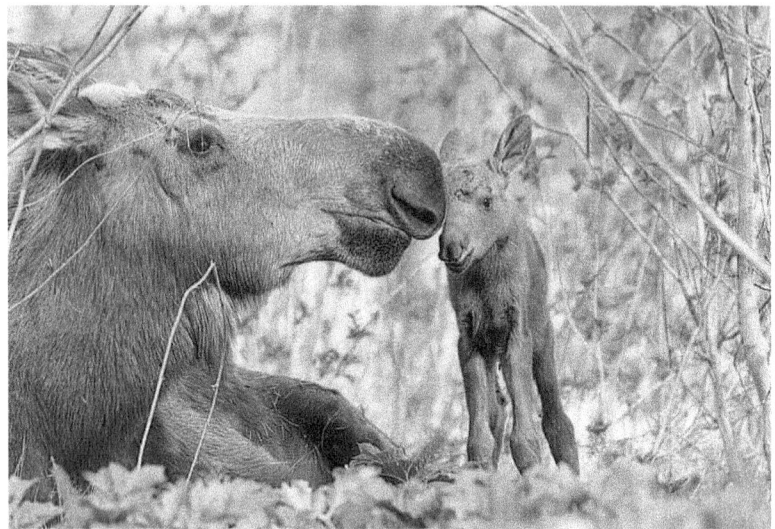

Mamma and Baby Moose. The moose of Alaska have allowed me to feel sheer joy, simply by just being in their presence. I can watch these amazing moose for hours. I still remain jealous of their beautiful eyelashes!

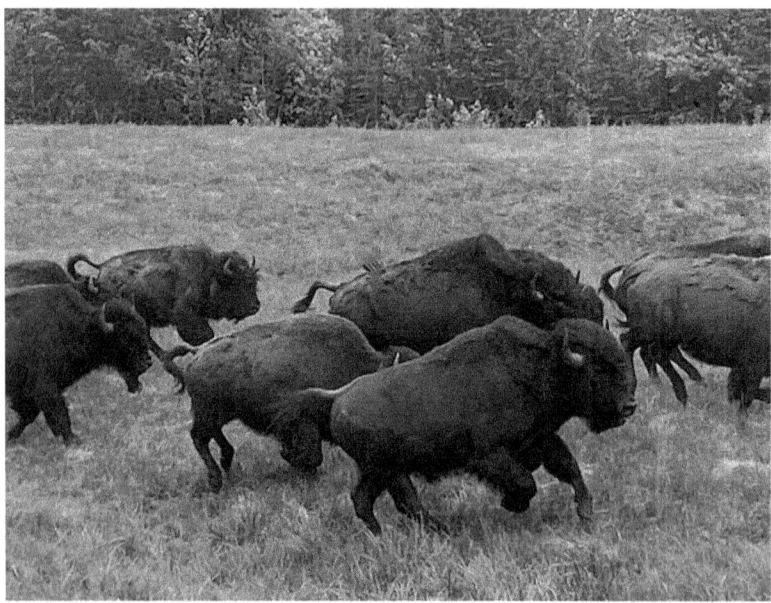

Always Strong, Like the Bison. How do we remain strong during these most challenging of times?

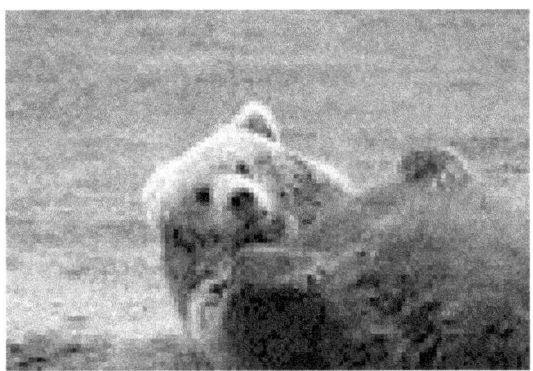
Bear Play. My deeply rooted heartfelt moment.

PART TWO
SITUATIONAL INSPIRATIONS

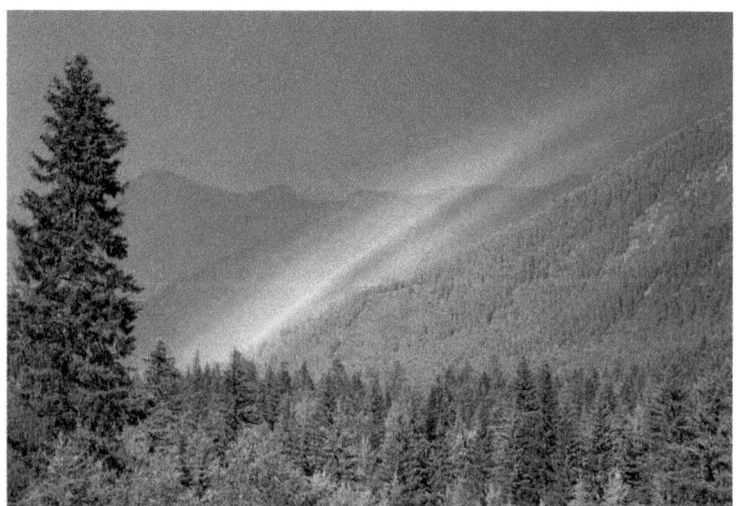

Rainbows. I love to stand still and just take in the awe of a rainbow. It reminds me to look toward the end of the rainbows during life's challenges.

Chapter 15
Everyone Feels Like the Only One

"The Times They Are A-Changing" Bob Dylan

Grand-parenting is different now. Grandparents of today remember their own childhoods, when their family schedules revolved around school and seeing their own aging grandparents, weekly, monthly, and always for holidays and birthdays. When did that change?

In my own family, Sundays used to be reserved for either driving long distances to our grandparent's house for dinner or hosting everyone at our suburban home for a Sunday BBQ. Grandparents were included as part of the family for all major events.

Today, we have many grandparents who feel forced to have a different mindset, partly by choice and partly because the times have changed. Absolutely every grandparent tells me, "I don't see my kids and grandchildren much". Parents and grandchildren today have very busy lives. Their grandchildren are growing up and moving forward with their own lives, which is how it should be, right?

Many who are now grandparents pushed themselves to exhaustion when they were parents; balancing family and career, all the while trying to meet the needs of both sets of aging parents and other relatives. We were a sandwich generation, meeting needs from both sides; our children and our aging parents. It was exhausting, yet we kept pushing, seldom making or allowing time for ourselves. We created this vision of running in circles and our children watched this. We didn't stop, we didn't relax, we failed to take time to just be or model that. Young parents and young families today are different. They do not want to live like that. Do you blame them?

Now our adult children are rising to the challenge of careers, more expensive mortgages, child care costs, and school loans, while keeping abreast of their child's cell phones and social media exchanges, to name just a few. Their children, unlike our children of yesteryear, are involved in sports, the arts, etc. Those activities are now more parent driven, no longer after school activities that include a bus ride home.

There is no longer a day to rest. Sunday's often include more sports practices, games, tournaments, recitals, cleaning up from the week that just ended and preparing for the week that is about to begin. It is exhausting to see how our adult children are running and running. If they are able, the few minutes they have in the week is to be able to work out so they can keep some semblance of sanity and health. Most of our families try so hard to find time to sit down and eat a meal together at night. With everyone on a different schedule, it remains a daunting task.

Social media and the constant demands on a cell phone cause a never- ending urgency that oftentimes results in anxiety. This is an anxiety many of us who are grandparents have not experienced in this way. So sometimes we feel forgotten, unimportant, not celebrated. It's so important now to reach out to these growing families, see how you can offer support, pick children up from an activity, prepare a meal. Perhaps, encourage a weekend getaway, so this exhausted couple can find a few minutes for themselves and perhaps each other.

Yes, it really is different today than when we were children or parents. Every grandparent feels like they are the only one who feels an increasing isolation, longing to be more involved. Sure, hearing their voices on a telephone call or seeing them on FaceTime is heartwarming. We miss them and don't know how to tell them that. Sometimes texting is all they can muster.

In conclusion, those of you who are grandparents; realize you are not alone, you all express the exact same thought. In conclusion, remember at the end of the day, even though times have changed, you really are loved, it just has a little different look.

Chapter 16
Truncated Grief

Have you ever had to deal with a type of grief that felt like it would never end? A grief that felt like it stayed within you every minute of every day? Will there ever be closure or must you live with this feeling of constant and frequent loss? We don't talk about this grief a lot. It is what I call a truncated grief; a grief that doesn't seem to have an end.

I have been thinking about truncated grief, a grief the world is feeling right now. Not only do we struggle with how to deal with the world around us, we struggle to know what to call it. First Co-Vid, then violence in Ukraine, unimaginable violence at now a new level in Israel. The amount of school and mass shootings has reached almost 400 and we are only half way through the year. That is more than one shooting a day. Many of us are faced with truncated grief that is consecutive and we must deal with the tangent fall outs that come with each new episode.

How do we navigate this truncation before it turns into anger, before it causes more isolation and divisiveness? So many of us are imploding. We are seeing the effects of those exploding?

To understand the trajectory of truncated grief is to attempt to cut it off. When we are in a state of truncated grief, we walk in circles, bleary eyed, not knowing what to think or how to organize moments in our lives. This leaves us without knowing what we should think within ourselves; let alone what to say to others.

What causes truncated grief, this constant state of gray? On a personal level, this could be as a result of a "bad divorce", the dispute that keeps on giving and becomes less about the child and more about each other. It could be mental health issues that keep our loved ones from us in a way we cannot control or fix. It could be when a child has been taken or has joined a gang or a cult. Truncated grief is often present when a parent becomes incarcerated, promising their child they are 'forever there' for them, yet they are not. It's when the words of the talk do not match their walk. These types of grief cannot be closed because they are caused by a different type of death. Often, there is a death of a relationship, the person we grieve is often not dead.

During these three years of Covid; our lives are forever changed. A strong person we love, may now be more limited in their ability to move around and take care of themselves. Many struggle with their ability to breathe. They may experience brain fog or extreme fatigue. The confidence with which we lived our days and ability to embrace the future with gusto, is now off balance. We are grieving a change in lifestyle without being able to close this circle of grief right now. Our hearts are forever changed, all of us are impacted by the atrocities we see around us.

While we witness and acknowledge the enormous strength and resilience we see by others all around the world, we grieve 'with them', 'for them', and 'for ourselves'; as we are well aware of the potential reach of everything surrounding us.

Should we talk about it this truncated grief with those around us? We acknowledge its presence, as there are just too many things to simply disconnect and say nothing. We cannot be complacent. While we may wish for all this shaky ground to simply go away on its own, we know it will not.

Many believe it is silence and avoidance that keeps equilibrium within our families and our community. If we don't talk about it, it will go away. In reality, it is the silence that actually feeds the grief. We think we are sparing our loved ones by keeping our feelings quiet within, maybe they won't notice. In reality, everyone is grieving. Start talking about the grief to better be able to support each other.

Truncated grief is horrible painful and is one of the biggest causes of anger and violence. Talk about it, ask questions, even when there are no answers. Just having the conversations are empowering to overcome truncated grief.

Chapter 17
Open Doors

"It takes courage to turn out to be who you really are." EE. Cummings

When life presents you with an open door, do you consider walking through it or walk right by? I've had many open doors throughout my life. Sometimes my decisions whether to walk through an open door had to be evaluated based on the timing or familial, financial, or career responsibilities.

There were a few times, I knew emphatically that I must walk through a door that was open in front of me, and I did so without hesitation. Now, today, I am compelled to look at these open doors through a different set of eyes. Is it because I am getting older, living through a pandemic, or the accumulation of personal tragedies? Maybe all of the above.

Reflecting, I have realized that when I have walked through many open doors in my life, they turned out to be amazing. When I have consciously permitted myself to release the feeling that I must have total control, life often happened better than the plan. I never would have predicted that the paths into my open doors would be so exciting and filled with unexpected possibilities and opportunities.

One of my favorite open doors occurred when I was walking down a hallway at my children's high school. I was asked to host an international exchange student for several weeks from Costa Rica. I asked when.

The teacher said "Tonight, the original family had to cancel hosting."

My response was absolutely! Walking through that single open door, allowed me to meet so many people and create such rich relationships, as well as offering the opportunity to work in this incredible country for eighteen years. I met spectacular people and was embraced into a culture of 'Pura Vida' (always life).

The cases I worked were challenging, intense, and what movies are made of. My partners and colleagues displayed great patience with me, as my master of Spanish is conversational and slang at best. I feel honored to have been a small part of training the professionals who opened the first juvenile prison. Previously, child does the crime, father does the time. Bridging methodology between crime labs in the United States and Costa Rica was moving and complex. I felt honored to be a part. To this day, I am thankful I walked through this open door. My friends and colleagues from Costa Rica always remain close in heart to both me and my family.

Now, I allow myself to appreciate the courage it takes to walk through the open doors in my life, a life which has been far more interesting than anything I could have planned. What is the most recent open door you have walked through?

Chapter 18
Circle of Estrangement

"To grow up, love doesn't just sit. It has to be remade all the time." Ursula K LeGuin

While the topic of estrangement is heartbreaking and isolating, it is one that 'almost' everyone I know lives with. Are our family ties becoming increasing estranged or is it something I just didn't recognize or understand as a child? Is the "do for me" mentality of the young asked of the older always been in play or are we seeing a new dynamic.

In my international travels, I have witnessed how respected and revered the older generations are. While the aging body may not be welcome, security of knowing you will be cared for and embraced by your family provided a layer of security as unwelcome life changes abound. Sometimes, the aging parents live with the youngest child. Sometimes they live with the oldest daughter. Each culture is different. Respect of our elders, parents, grandparents was understood even here in the United States until….I'm not sure when, but it changed.

The sense of duty, loyalty, respect, and responsibility of our parents is not guaranteed anymore. Sometimes, I hear the demeaning way an adult child speaks to their aging parent and it is with disrespect and condescension. Sometimes, they won't talk to them at all. Oftentimes, aging parents tell me their texts are not answered. There are countless aging who tell me they are heartbroken as they never would have treated heir parents the way they are treated. Some feel badly they raised their children with such entitlement, there is blatant disregard.

I have recently read an article about entitlement, ….. addressing the issue that adult children today are angrier at their parents. The author of that article suggesting apologies should be offered from the aging parent for all the mistakes they made while raising their child.

I'd like to offer another spin on estrangement. First, the image of everyone sitting down to weekly Sunday dinner such as shown on Blue Bloods is not the norm. We might like it to be, but it is not. Adult children, raising our grandchildren are pushed to the brink of busy. While we might like to see them and talk to them more, their days are filled with so many demands professionally and personally, there are times I do not comprehend how they manage all the demands.

Of course, it feels better when everyone is together and gets along but our means of comparing how life should be now between the generations is challenging. This circle of estrangement is causing an increase in loneliness, depression. And a sadness that permeates life.

What is saddest to me, what we should be cherishing the most during these difficult times feels like it is going away; family. Family connections and the richness that comes full circle feels like it is greatly diminishing at a time when it is most needed. Knowing about….

*What was your life like growing up?
*What kind of work did your parents and grandparents do?
*What was it like living through a war during your life?
*What were your dreams?
*Tell me about my parents when they were growing up?
*Who do I seem the most like in our family and why?
*What is your favorite memory of me?
*What was the best decade of your life?
*How do you want me to remember you?

If you can't talk to your children and grandchildren about these important questions; then write down the answers collectively and send it to them or save it for them. One day, when you are not around, they will want to know the answers to these questions. I know this to be true.

Twice in my life, I have been told I was going to die. Doctors were hopeful, but uncertain if I would survive. The first time my children were very young; only nine, seven and one years old. The thought of not watching them grow up was sheer agony me for me. As I thought about their childhood, I was deeply saddened they would never know me and about their lives and mine. So, I bought each one of them a chest and started collecting all the things that were so rich and important from their lives. I neatly packaged them in their chest; the little outfit I brought each home from the hospital wearing, the handprints they made in pre-school, and so much more. I bought each of them a journal with a lovely, personally chosen cover and wrote them everything I feared I might not be able to say. It didn't change the diagnosis, but it did change my steps as I walked down each path.

One day they will wish they had more time with you. There will be so many questions they have to ask you. They are presently unaware of how much they would love just one more hour to have a conversation and embrace you for one more hug. Give them this most valuable gift now. It will enrich both them and you; as you enjoy this most private of moments with the children you cherish.

Chapter 19
We Are Dedicated Professionals

"Those who bring sun to the lives of others, cannot keep it from themselves." J. M. Barrie

Are you a first responder, a teacher, a counselor, a social worker, or a nurse? Do you have a loved one away in the military? We are walking into the holidays; one of the most challenging times of the year.

Professionally, December has always been the month with the most callouts, the most agitation, the month when many around me have a short fuse. We feel like we are supposed to be merry and bright. Isn't that what we are told about this time of the year? The images of families gathering around the table in perfect harmony is not necessarily what our realities are. While traditions seem sweet, the world does not feel like it is in a festive place right now. Our reality feels like everything around us is discombobulated.

Adding to this, the work we do is difficult, on so many levels. During these distorted and dystopian times, it feels even more so. Many around us are angry. Their voices are angry. Their posturing is angry. Their tone and facial expressions are angry. Oftentimes, they force a smile they do not feel.

It is confusing to try to modulate the situations in front of us. Some days, there is little that makes sense. More and more people around us seem to be crumbling, reaching out to us; desperate for our words of wisdom, soothing words that will magically change the course of their day, their week. We give all we can, but that is getting more and more difficult.

I appreciate the challenges we face as dedicated professionals. We are always there to help others, yet oftentimes, we struggle ourselves. No matter how much we try to take care of ourselves, the mountain can be a steep climb.

Numbing is rough. Feeling is rough. It's so hard to reconcile the best ways to navigate our work and private lives in these challenging times. We give it everything we've got to stay attuned; attuned to our family, our friends, our clients, our jobs. Some days, it seems to get more challenging, other days less so. I truly understand the push and pull of needing to feel the humanity around us without becoming totally depleted. We have unique situations that many cannot conceptualize.

So how do we move forward in this most challenging time? How do we restore ourselves? We start by looking for an ever so slight moment of joy in the day, making sure to really 'see' the joy that restores our soul. Some call it glimmers.

We look up in the sky and follow the movement of a cloud or breathe in the painting of the stars in the sky. We look at our most favorite animal, and take in their incredible ability to live in the moment. And when something is funny, really funny, we laugh from deep within our belly, even if we are all alone.

We can grant ourselves permission to nurture ourselves, something we are not used to doing. Cook that favorite food reserved for the most special of times. And when you are in physical pain, acknowledge it, touch it, rub it with lotion and acknowledge that pain. Tap your body to feel your own movement and flow.

If all that doesn't work, turn the lights off, lay on the floor; palms faced down for grounding. Take some slow breaths, imagine the most beautiful place you have ever seen, and tell yourself that in this moment, you are good.

This is exactly what I do to help me navigate through the most unimaginable of cases and the roughest patches in my life. I imagine the snow- capped mountains and the glistening blue water.

My coat and boots are already packed!

Chapter 20
Who's Running Your House?"

"I know my child hangs around with other kids who do drugs, but my child doesn't do drugs." SLM

I've yet to have a parent say, "Sue, life is great, come for coffee. Instead, they contact me regarding these similar thematic issues:

*My child is at the fork of the road and I'm afraid they are heading down a bad path. I am worried about the friends they are hanging around with.

*I'm afraid of my child. She/he is abusive, even hitting me. I am embarrassed to admit this.

*My daughter is hanging with a "bad boy, she is going to get caught up in some bad things going down as an accomplice.

*My adult child has graduated, but won't look for a job, help around the house, sleeps all day or plays video games."

*My child's grades are plummeting and I don't know what to do."

*My child is a victim of cyberbullying, and I am afraid he/she is going to kill himself/herself."

*My child seems totally unmotivated except for social media. We have absolutely no conversation."

*My child is on the cell phone non-stop. I don't get more than 2 word responses.

Sometimes, these calls even come from grandparents raising their grandchildren at a time in their lives when they were hoping to take life a little easier, but now have the responsibility of supporting young children.

Welcome to my world as a criminologist. It has been a rather unique career, one that emulated as a sign of the times, not a planned career. I love the families I work with. I have the privilege to know them at the darkest time of their lives and be part of the journey as they walk out the other side. Some of these families are facing some horrific realities. I've been working with them for over thirty-five years in various settings; in their homes, schools, community centers, in prison, and on the streets.

I can relate to most of these kids. I was one of them a long time ago. With the help of some amazing professionals, some good luck, and grabbing on to the hands that reached out to me, I've had a successful career working with extremely high risk youth, violent, and angry people and their families. In the course of my work, I develop strategies to bring about positive change for youth and families, training professionals throughout the USA and internationally.

These families are just like you and me. These are parents who love their kids. They work hard and try to do right by them. Most are not neglectful. Sometimes they are doing everything right, but the child's behaviors are a result of experiences outside the family unit. These parents come from all professional backgrounds, all socio-economic levels, some have experienced divorce, some have dealt with the death, the challenges of blended families, or mental health within the family.

Some live in beautiful homes, some do not. Most are trying to make it through the day the best they can. They want to enjoy their children for the remaining years they still live at home. How old are the children these parents call me about? Some, are as young as six, others as old as twenty-eight. Why 28? Many children are remaining home or returning.

Why does a parent call me? They cannot change their chaos, unpredictability, and roller coasting. Their lives are filled with negativity, disrespect, and violence. They are afraid; for themselves and afraid for their children.

These parents feel like they have lost control of their house. When I ask them "Who's running your house?", they all have the same answer. "Not me! My child is running the house and I want the power back!" Some feel their child has been so traumatized by outside influences, it has affected the family in a profound way. If none of this applies to you, consider yourself lucky. That is not the case with most families today. It is not solely the parents who are raising their children these days, so who is: social media, network and streamed media, video games, and friends? In many cases, parents are in the last position here.

YOU can take the power back! YOU can say No! YOU do not want to be their best friend until adulthood. YOU can take a locked door off the hinge! Most importantly, YOU can and should, look in their room; privacy is not a right, it's a privilege! YOU are the parent and YOU are running the house!

Chapter 21
Averting the Shoot

"Never let a problem to be solved be more important than a person to be loved."

Thomas S. Monsoon

I have averted and worked the aftermath of school shootings throughout the United States and internationally. It is a complex issue that is growing out of control. School shootings have a deeper precipice than gun control and mental health issues. I believe addressing only those two issues alone will be a diversion, not a solution.

There are two commonalities in absolutely ALL the cases I have accepted involving "school shootings". All the shooters shared a background of trauma which they endured along with a lack of connectedness towards others. This is a common thread amongst all the shooters, no exception.

There are many children and teenagers all around us who are experiencing chronic, complex trauma. We are looking right at them, but we do not see them. Nor do we see the enormous pain in their eyes.

Start looking at these children and see them. Is there a lack of congruence between their eyes and their face? Is there a lack of congruence between their eyes and their body language? Are their eyes sad? Do they display pain? Are they faking a smile? When there is a lack of congruence, always believe the eyes.

Pay particular attention to dead eyes. Trauma is what you are looking to identify. Initially, you don't need to know the details or analyze them, just identify that a teen appears to be struggling. Oftentimes, many young people in trauma will retreat inward. For some, their rage escalates.

Next, they find groups to identify with on social media, who validate the commonality of their feelings. They may 'follow' and read about all the shooters who have come before them, aspiring to be like them or even more 'grandiose'. None of the potential shooters I have worked with had a mental health diagnosis which would have identified them during a background check. It doesn't mean they didn't have mental health issues, it means it would not have come up on a check because this information was not in the system.

The Uvalde shooter, like every shooter before him, gave out warning signs. Those around him either didn't see it, didn't believe it, or didn't know what to do. I get calls from parents, young people, and professionals that they fear a student's plan for a shoot is imminent. We avert that by working with the youth, family, and sometimes staff and community to ensure innocents are not killed.

The trajectory of these potential mass shootings can be averted when just one person is attuned to the warning signs of trauma, potential violence, and rage. Then....they must find the fortitude and courage to speak up, even if they fear they may be wrong or cannot process what they are seeing could potentially be a reality.

Occasionally, someone does speak up to be met with a deaf ear or the recipient doesn't know what to do. As a society, we erroneously believe if we identify a youth, fix them with a prescription for ADHD or depression, then we have done enough. In terms of school violence there are many more layers and medicating is not a quick fix.

What's the answer? Start training more interventionists; a person who a youth with trauma can learn to connect with and trust. We must teach strategies to connect with these kids, and bring them to a calmer place. Connections! This is the missing piece!

*Once they are de-escalated, they can be referred to a counselor so the that cycle of trauma can be broken. There is the misperception that rage must be observable screaming, while many with rage are actually raging deep within. For many of the young people and families I work with, the trauma and rage are deep rooted. Sometimes, youth may appear detached or lack reality. Are we looking at a mental health disorder or a behavioral disorder? Has the youth been identified with oppositional defiant disorder or conduct disorder? These are the questions we should be asking. Simply using the phrase 'more mental health needed' without learning about and identifying specifics will be a band aide at best.

The most important strategy is to explore whether a young person is connected to anyone or anything. Then look at what is missing, not just what is present This is the reality of my work as a criminologist. Initially, I am with a family for many consecutive hours or days at a time in order to connect with the youth and their family. My goal is to bring their entire situation to place of calm. I'm still with them continually for hours and days after that. Then we refer the youth and or family to a counselor or therapist.

In conclusion, the lens we need to start looking through is so much more than gun control and a Red Flag Law. It is about learning about interventions and doing better as a society to make connections with youth, families and respond to them when they have a potentially violent youth in their home. The trauma that some young people are struggling with every day can forever change the trajectory of so many who come in their path. Trauma prohibits the ability to engage in normal life cycles and we need to recognize that. Simply and solely changing gun laws and hiring more mental health professionals are not the impetus of what is needed. We need to start engaging more with each other, be more present in each other's lives, and be kind to one another. These are a few steps to breaking the cycle of trauma so another disengaged and angry teenager doesn't enter a school and shoot innocent students and teachers or the president.

Chapter 22
The Code of Secrecy

"The most important thing in communication is hearing what isn't said." Peter Trucker

Are you the child of an incarcerated parent? Do you know someone who has an incarcerated parent in their past? Do you know someone who has or has had a parent on parole or probation? I am sure you do, even if you are not aware of who they are. These children are an 'invisible population'. Oftentimes, most people have no idea who they are; whether they are all grown up or still youthful.

As a criminologist, I have worked with inmates and their children for decades; in prison and on the outside, during and after. There has been an uptick of interest in a book, "Voices of Children of Incarcerated Parents. It has become my best-selling book recently. We are talking about almost twelve million children across the United States.

These children live with a big secret and often live in a type of trauma that most around them are unaware of. Even though our rates of incarceration continue to grow, little attention has been given to the children of incarcerated parents. Oftentimes, we have no idea who they are. Should we?

Most incarcerated parents return to our communities eventually. They get out, they are parents and our neighbors. Many are on parole or probation. The dynamic is always the same. Inmates seldom discuss their children with professionals who work in the system.

Criminal justice professionals often ask the right questions. In some cases, investigative reports are given to judges, prior to sentencing. These reports may or may not include information about their children. Some pre-trial and sentenced institutions ask inmates if they have children.

Incarcerated parents seldom respond affirmatively. Instead they may share they have lost all contact with their family and they leave it at that. Sometimes, this is true. Sometimes it is not.

As a criminologist, they tell me they have many children, some have seven and some have close to fifteen. What is the reason for this "code of secrecy" about their children?

The answer is two- fold. First, the family has decided to keep news of the parent's incarceration private. That part of their lives is kept "behind the door". The children do not divulge to their teachers, counselors, not even to their friends. The reason is fear. The custodial parent and their family do not know how they will be received within the community once their secret is revealed. Many find it easier to simply not discuss the incarcerated parent.

Secondly, many do not divulge because they don't want interaction with their state's child protective services agency. In most cases, the child remains with a family member during the term of parental incarceration. That might be the other parent. It is frequently the grandparent. To an incarcerated parent, this is the next best option for their child. If they cannot raise their child, they prefer a family member step in, as opposed to the foster care system. The biggest fear for an incarcerated parent is the state will step in and remove their children.

If that happens, life takes on an entirely different look. The family will be required to follow certain rules and be accountable to the state for many aspects of the child's life; counseling sessions, possible medication, inspections of the family home, etc. In some states, an incarcerated parent's rights may be severed during a window of twenty-two months if they cannot regain physical custody. Some believe children of incarcerated parents are automatically under the auspices of child protective services, receiving counseling to deal with their parent's crime, incarceration, visiting, and even re-entry. This is not necessarily true.

In my experience, most are surprised to learn children of incarcerated parents are not involved with services. There is a surge in the number of grandparents raising grandchildren, without any assistance. That is because few people actually think about children of incarcerated parents at all. Thus, the circle of secrecy continues, as these families navigate their altered lifestyle, day by day, alone.

The next factor always weighing heavy on children of an incarcerated parent is whether to 'Visit or Not Visit the Parent in Prison'. Would you?

Chapter 23
What Do Children with an Incarcerated Parents Look Like?

"I'm always here for you, baby, behind the bars! But you cannot call me, you cannot touch me. Always remember, I'm here for you." SLM

Children of an incarcerated parents have unique characteristics. Most will present as overachievers working hard not to follow in their parent's footsteps. Not the picture you initially visualized? They are faced with tremendous trauma during various stages of their parent's incarceration. Initially, they have to find a way to reconcile, within themselves, about the crime their parent has committed. If the crime is infamous, the child sees the story of their parent's crime over and over on the news.

In this early stage, many try to handle themselves stoically at school and in their community. They are aware others are scrutinizing them. Will they be judged by the actions of their parent? If they have a girlfriend, "Will she break up with me?"

The child is often distracted and pre-occupied during the course of their school day, ruminating over unanswered questions. Why didn't the parent think about this before committing the crime?

They worry about their parent's safety inside prison. They feel mixed emotions of anger, sadness, confusion, betrayal, frustration, and exhaustion. Often, they do not sleep well at night, feeling unsettled, unable to reconcile the turmoil of emotions. They keep this to themselves not wanting to create more stress in the house.

The judicial process is a nebulous time as the trial can take over two years. This is the 'gray time', the unknown. Some children are forced to move, downsizing or with grandparents.

Look at all the grandparents raising their grandchildren. Why? Their plans of retirement put on hold, their finances are stretched beyond their budget, and many divorce their new spouse, given ultimatums about raising their biological grandchildren. Today's changing values bring even more of a conundrum. Should a new boyfriend come to the door or beep? One hundred dollars for a pair of jeans, uh, No! Social media and curfews are other causes for disparity.

Once the trial or a plea agreement is over, the incarcerated parent settles into a sentenced correctional facility. This is the calmest time for all since there's more routine. The "new family" adjusts and learns how to dance in their new life.

Family cannot call the prison to speak with an inmate. So, the family never waits for that inmate call each day. Sometimes it comes and sometimes it does not. Calls are usually restricted to fifteen minutes.

Children can write letters or draw pictures, no paint, markers, colored pencils accepted. If not within guidelines, the drawing is returned. Some children are not aware of these regulations. They sent daddy a picture, it was returned. Drugs laced within the markers or paint created this rule.

Who discusses this with child? Most people have no idea about the regulations that lead to frustration and self-esteem issues for the child. There are no guide books for children of an incarcerated parent. The family walks through this experience blindly.

"To visit or not to visit a parent in prison", a complex issue. These visits require long trips and lots of waiting, an overwhelming experience for anyone. Who prepares the child to hear the "Chang-Chang" of the heavy metal doors of the sally ports? Who prepares them for the visual of seeing so many inmates in one place.

There are strict rules for all visitors for a reason. Who explains this to the child? Sometimes visits are through glass, sometimes over a computer screen. Who explains why they cannot touch mommy or sit on daddy's lap?

Broken promises are devastating. During visits, the incarcerated parent makes detailed promises about how wonderful life is going to be when they get out. Possible frustrations in anticipation of re-integration is seldom discussed; family dynamics, finances, jobs. A parent's release is one of the more tumultuous times. They should be excited their parent is going to return. Instead, they feel conflicted.

Who debriefs the prison visit with the child? Who answers all the questions the child has about the prison? No one. Many cannot sleep the night after a visit.

Who are these children? They are all around you. Look and you will see them. This is my final piece about children of incarcerated parents. For more information, my book Reunification of Incarcerated Parents With Their Children in Amazon & Kindle, under my name.

Chapter 24
Are You Afraid of Your Child?

"You are not alone! This is my number one callout."
SLM

Are you afraid of your child? Do you secretly worry that one day you may die at the hands of your child? This is the "other domestic violence" few will talk about. It is my number one call out. If one of your friends were afraid of their child, how would you know?

For some, this story will resonate with you. For others, thank goodness it doesn't. To be able to vocalize this fear takes a long time. First, comes the self-rationalizing that you, the parent, must be seeing your child incorrectly. Let's give it a little more time and your 'imagination' will surely change. Then it doesn't. Who do you talk to about this type of domestic violence? Will you be criticized for being irrational or being a poor parent? So many fears keep this painful secret hidden deep within.

Until the day, when this cannot be hidden anymore because suddenly you are locking the outside of your child's bedroom door when everyone goes to sleep at night or locking your own door. You hide all the knives in your house-just in case. Some parents find themselves deliberately planning not to be home alone with their child, especially as their child gets into their teen years. Excuse after excuse is made within the parent's mind until one defining incident, usually a physical altercation. The child may hit the parent, punch them, try to strangle them or whack them with an object. They may threaten to harm then over and over. I have been called for hundreds of these situations over the years. And it is not necessarily both parents who are the targeted victims, it can be only one parent and one sibling. All my cases have the same theme and follow the same trajectory.

By the time a parent calls me, this cycle has gone on for quite a while. It takes everything the parent has in them to be able to share their situation with me. They ruminate over what they did wrong. Usually, the other children in the family don't act this way. What to do? Many parents are afraid to tell others about this horror for added fear that other families won't want to hang around with them anymore, or they fear they will be judged in other avenues of their lives, such as professionally. Instead, they stay quiet secretly praying for their child to hurry up, grow up, and leave their house.

Adult children abuse their parents as well. I see the parents walking on eggshells in their own homes, never able to find peace. Adult children are living at home longer now or returning home in higher numbers than previous generations, thus the cycle continues. Oftentimes, it is a minor comment that the parent makes which triggers the explosive behaviors. The parent will do anything to keep their child from blowing up. Many work hard to avoid telling their child 'NO', as this too is a predictable trigger. Some of the parents who have frequently witnessed these explosive behaviors, come to recognize the initial signs of imploding. This gives them time to leave their house or leave the room. Sometimes the parent finds themselves soft stepping around their child to make sure everything remains copasetic.

If I am able to work with this child before they are seventeen, it is possible for me to turn this situation around. Later, strategies look differently; simply because the child now has the potential to be involved with the adult legal system. In most states, domestic violence calls are known to be one of the most dangerous of all call outs. Usually it requires that one of the participants be taken into custody. Oftentimes, I see the parent identified and detained when in actuality, it is the child who was violent.

Who are these parents? They are executives of companies, educated professionals, they are the people standing in line with you at the grocery store or ordering a latte next to you. As we acknowledge October as Domestic Violence Month, don't forget to acknowledge the "other domestic violence".

First step? Are you open to someone sharing this type of domestic violence experience with you? If you are not, the parent who is a victim can sense this and will not speak of their situation with you.

Chapter 25
Climbing Steep Mountains

"When I am climbing the steepest mountains, I build my strength." SLM

"I will not live my life with extreme stress; personally, and professionally at the same time. One must balance the other, to stay mentally healthy. I would not have been able to stay in the game otherwise."

I have believed these two "things" for as long as I can remember. It is the only way I've been able to survive as a criminologist. While people are running away from rage and violence, I run into chaos. I identify and de-escalate to prevent further harm and violence. I am referred to as a zero- level responder. My number one call out is the "other domestic violence" when a young person tries to hurt or kill their parent(s). My second most frequent call out involves school shootings or violence when a young person has created plans to commit a school shoot or violence; not yet carried out. There is a moment in time to turn this situation, so it does not end in tragedy. I have other cases, but these are my most frequent.

There is one commonality amongst my cases; someone involved is under 28 years old. Often, I work with first responders. I am grateful for these amazing men and women.

They, too, live by these two premises to build inner strength and work hard to stay mentally healthy. Today, we include "Front Liners", Teachers, Administrators, Counselors, Mental Health Therapists, Nurses, Doctors, College Professors, Social Workers to our list of heroes.

Last week.. yesterday, more shootings in which the suspects are fifteen to eighteen years old. Another youth remanded into the adult system for heinous crime. We are saddened, not shocked, increasingly numb to these events. Juvenile waiver/youth remand. Difficult as it was for me to see such extreme violence perpetrated by sixteen year olds over the decades, it was rare, the professional part of my life. I was able to modulate because it wasn't around me all the time.

According to the Gun Violence Archives, as of last week there were more than 531 mass shootings in the United States this year. The days of extreme violence being my narrow scope is now happening at insurmountable rates in our personal life as well.

How has this happened? I must clear my head constantly with exercise and music to sweat out the insanity and comprehend the enormity. I have thousands of followers and friends who are first responders and front liners. We are all looking for answers, for support, to maintain strength and sound mental health. Overall, the lack of attunement and disengagement is astronomical. Many still believe it is the kid from the "over there" with the real problems. That could not be more incorrect and short sighted. It is your child, my child, our child. We are ALL exhausted trying to make it in an ever-changing world. We acknowledge that most around us are good people, trying to be good parents, good community members. But now, coming home to our children and families requires more understanding, along with a constant vigilance, on top of our mounting exhaustion.

A new reality; the screen, holds the attention of our young people, yet conversely, it keeps them more disengaged, prohibiting them from interacting with each other in a humane way. Their new reality is what is on the other end of that screen. It determines their confidence, empowerment, and for some the trajectory of their future. Parents and professionals cannot keep up! Add a pandemic, now we are all forever changed, a culture surrounded in trauma, rage, and violence. And no one knows what to do because we can't step off the merry-go around.

Strength breeds change; change breeds strength? Now, I need to add yet another "third thing" to maintain that balance I have embraced all my life. Now two is not enough. I'm going to work out now, to keep good mental health, and clear my head, hoping to find my third "thing" for these new times. I will be back at it tomorrow with a clear head.

Chapter 26
Waiting for The Normal

"Happiness Takes Courage", written by my teacher
Paul Berbaum , spoken by Jon Hamm

What an absolutely unique time in history this is! We are all sitting on the edge of our seats waiting, just waiting for our lives to "return to normal". We are doing everything we can think of to circumvent the many changes that have plagued our young people, families, professionals and communities. Heck, we are waiting for our nation and the world to return to normal.

Individually, we are surviving by putting one foot in front of the other, mindfully replaying the saying "carpe diem" (seize the day). But at the end of the day, at the end of the week, we are exhausted and privately scared how the future is going to look. I've seen this present in two ways; denial of what is happening around us, a type of dystopian / distorted lack of reality or a hyper charged anger that seems to be boiling just below the surface of people's skin. Anxiety, anger, poor manners and the acceptance of muddy character is the result of both. There is this frenetic energy that seems to be thick in the air, I almost feel like I can grab it.

We all feel like we are going through hell alone as we are waiting for the normal to return. Social media would have us believe everyone is thriving with happiness and traveling the world. This makes us feel like we are the only one's struggling. "What is wrong with me" is the intrinsic message we keep playing over and over inside ourselves. What can we do as we wait for the normal to return?

I've always prided myself on being grounded and balanced; it has been my lifelong foundation. Balance between the work and the home, balance between the good and the bad, balance between the have and have not, balance between the right and wrong. Now, it is more difficult to find the balance as the lines blur without any respite. The grounding is getting more difficult as the life feels like it is shaking all around us.

Frustrations are growing. Our Lack of attunement is expanding. The basics in life are more stressful than they have ever been. People's character appears to be similar to that in a bad movie; one we would prefer not to watch. Children go to school scared, go in their bedrooms and connect to screens that either create a lack of reality or further cement fear and uncertainty. What's the answer? Perhaps, we are in the new normal now and must learn to springboard from the reality we are in. We don't have the luxury now to wait for our normal to return. In doing this, we are losing time, living life in a blur and absorbing a total lack of reality which is slowly weighing us down.

As a criminologist, in my professional life; I am used to a lack of reality, stepping over blurred lines, and marginal character. Now, what used to be exclusively my professional life working with crime, is commonplace; in my community. My new normal, your new normal… Where do we go from here?

Step One: Acknowledge the reality. Nothing will change if we don't acknowledge the problem.

Step Two: Get healthy, get strong, take care of what's around you-don't look the other way. And this is how we respond to life in the new normal. Complacently waiting for the return of 'yester-year' is no longer an option.

Print this out. Put it in your time capsule to bury for the next fifty years. Then our grandchildren and great-grandchildren will get a sense of how we embraced the creation of what is most certainly, our new normal.

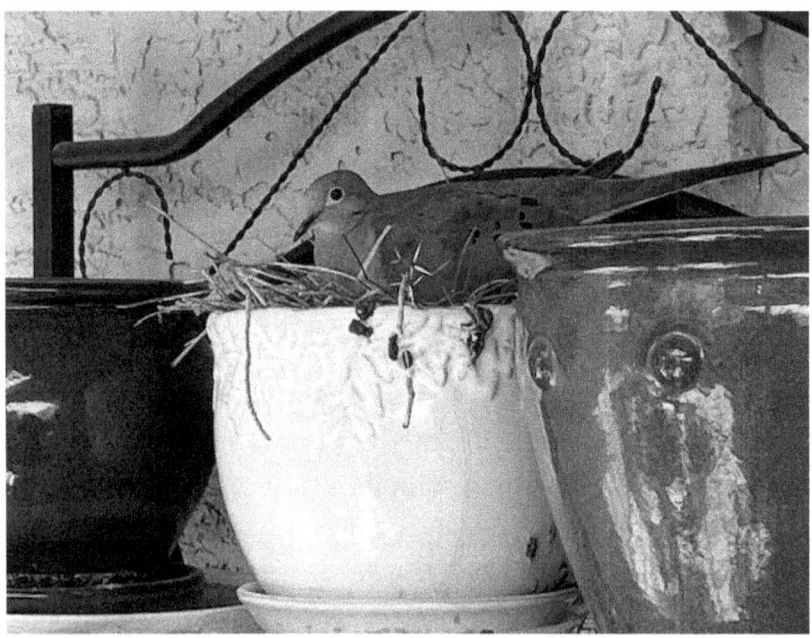

Paloma de Paz and Her Babies. Every year, I find great joy when the Doves of Peace lay their eggs in our flower pots. Every morning, I go out to them and say "Good morning" and every evening, I tell them, "Good night."

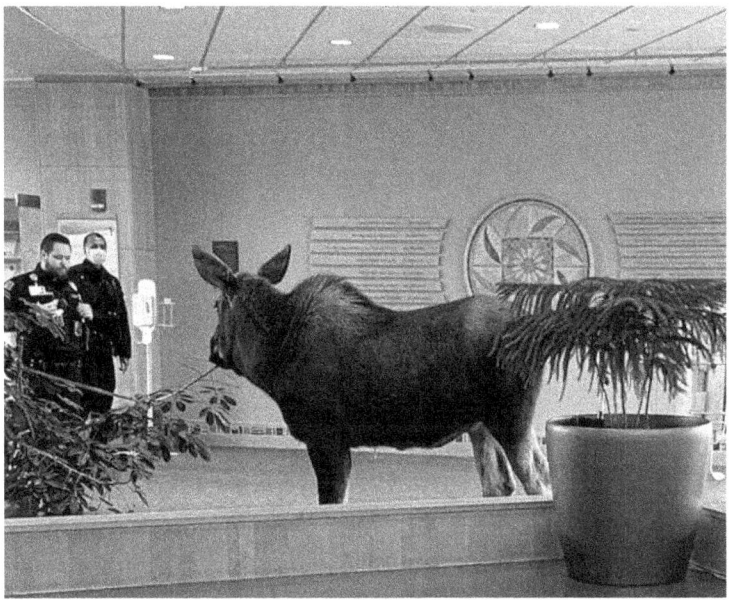

Moose in the Lobby. True Story. Only an Alaskan is not surprised by a moose in a hospital lobby. Thank you to our law enforcement officers as they navigate what became a national story!

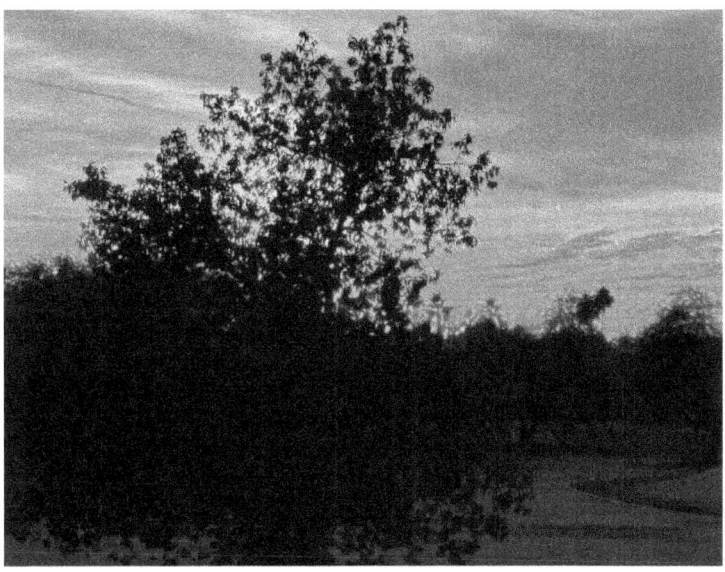

The Sun Will Rise and Set Tomorrow. Remember this on those challenging days

The Book Of Heartfelt Moments

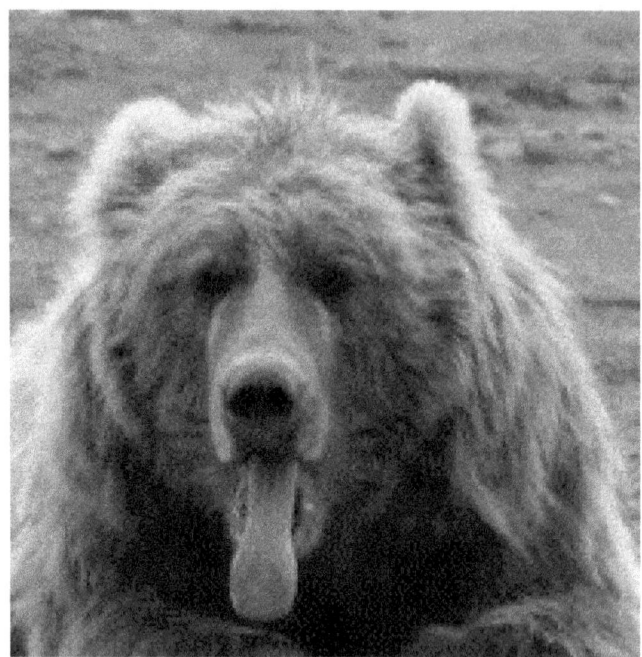

It's Been A Rough Day: I took this picture on a photography trip to Katmai with my husband. I am moved by the strength, instinct and wisdom of 'the Bear'.

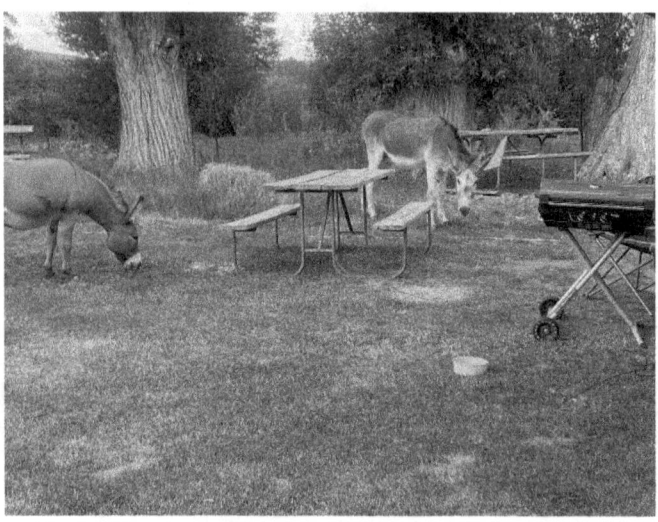

Camping with the Donkeys. Thank you Colorado for the forever memory of camping with the donkeys

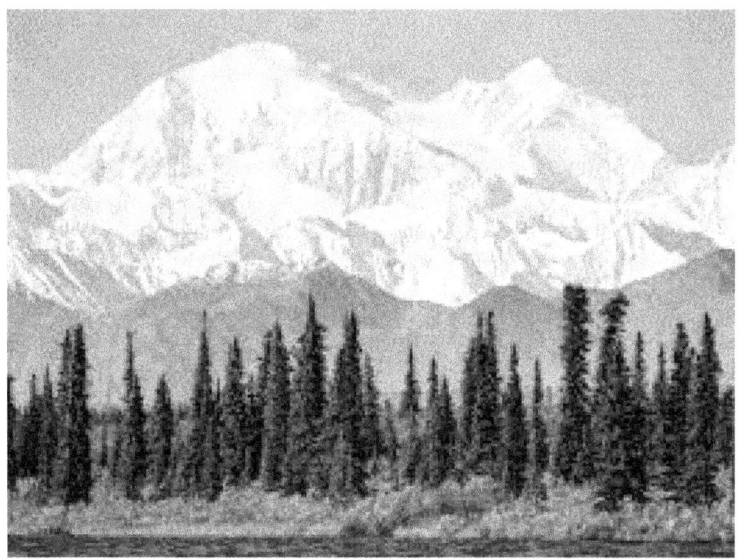

Feeling the Home. The gift of waking up each day to see the snow capped mountains of Alaska puts life in perspective. The images of mountainous grandeur are deep within, always reminiscent of home.

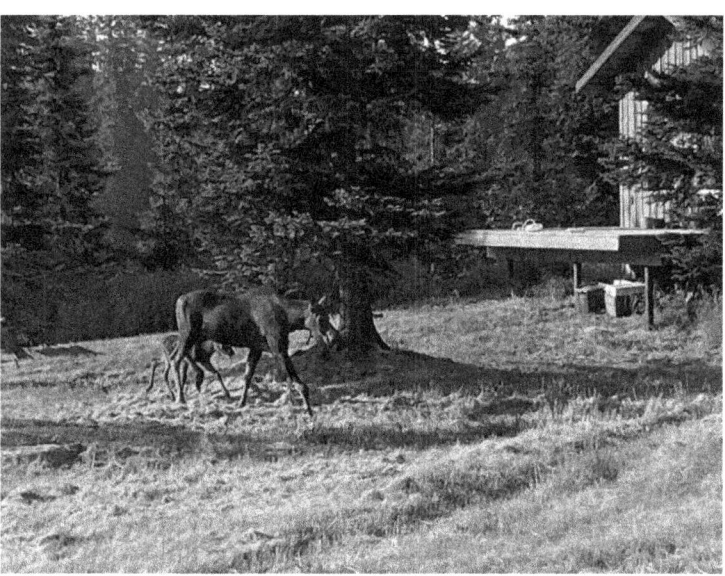

Moose Point. She throws her calf at Baby Moose Point, then takes him for a walk to introduce him to the land.

Epilogue

Today, I had a call that filled me up. It reminded me that chaotic and disconcerting as our times are right now, there are amazing young people out there, who are compassionate and moved to make a difference in the world around them.

This young lady read my book 'Reunification of Incarcerated Parents and Children'. I wrote that book over twelve years ago. She processed the plight of these children and families chapter by chapter. She thoughtfully tried to understand all that ensconced the lifestyle of marginalized children, who live life with a secret; fearful they will be shunned by the deeds of their incarcerated parent. She was moved by this topic because it is still one of the few that is seldom spoken about.

Calling me from across the country, she initially spoke softly gaining confidence as our time together grew. I applauded her courage and maturity to reach out to an author, wanting to learn more about this taboo subject. She wanted to know what my motivation was to write this book. Thoughtfully, processing my responses, she navigated the journey that affects millions upon millions of children.

This young woman displayed something I don't see or write about much with youth, she shared passion and voice. Sharing her voice gave her strength and it gave me hope that there can, and will be, a generation coming forth who wants to make a difference. We also talked about being a woman in the field of criminology stressing the importance of support; support by those around you, to lift you up in a world that would sometimes like to un-invite you.

We spoke about her outstanding parents who are raising a daughter with so much passion and conviction, a daughter who advocates for causes that impact young people. To raise a child today, who is curious about the world and cares for others, is challenging these days. To yearn to know more and provide space to make a difference in the lives of others, at such a young age, is even more uncommon. Well done, mom and dad.

And she closed with a question. She wondered if she could share some of the strategies to de-escalate anger and problem solve with other teens she knew.

After our time together ended, she sent me an email thanking me for helping her understand children of incarcerated parents and thanking me for helping her with the future projects she will be creating from our time together. She wrote her work will be 'amazing because of me'. What humility, a quality we don't see much today. I wrote her back and shared her projects will be amazing because of her, her voice, and her courage. What a gift for me to see a young person with so much passion to help others.

She told me my book provided her an avenue to look at her future working with social injustices and causes which affect children. She read my book and it may create a path for her life. This is not unlike the book I read when I was twelve years old, 'The Kitty Genovaisse Story'. Reading that book set me on a path to be a criminologist, at a time when I was grounded in my room for a month, for even considering such a profession as a woman. That book changed my life. I followed my passion and my voice to work with crime focusing on children. Could my book move another young woman in the same way I was moved? I had never thought about that before, until today.

I will continue to embrace these heartfelt moments around me as a way of getting through these challenging times. Today, I feel full, recognizing that not only will the sun rise and set tomorrow, but it will be a good day, because of the young people who aspire to make a difference in this chaotic and sometimes unforgiving world we now live in.

About Author

When people are running away from rage and violence, Susan Magestro's unique, thirty-five-year career has evolved in to one of running into the chaos.

Susan Magestro, criminologist, interventionist, international presenter and university instructor is now returning to writing full time. As a former newspaper columnist and author, she is excited to be merging her two passions; the world of criminology and writing.

Susan has written five books.
- 'Empowering the Victim: New Approaches to Stopping Bullying' (2009)
- 'Reunification of Incarcerated Parents With Their Children and Families' (2016)
- 'Raging From Within: De-Escalating Angry People' (2021)
- 'Voices From the Box' (2023)
- 'Breaking the Cycles of Trauma: Through A Daughter's Eyes' (2024)
- 'The Book of Heartfelt Moments" (2024)

Coming in 2025, the psychological thriller, 'Priscilla Breen, Criminologist"
- Book One: 'Capture'

www.ingramcontent.com/pod-product-compliance
Lightning Source LLC
Chambersburg PA
CBHW071721020426
42333CB00017B/2352